The Secret Knowledge of Yoga

An introduction and guide for practice

By Aaron Brachfeld

for Gauri

i had no intention to benefit others when i wrote this
Merely to familiarize my own mind
For it is by familiarity that confidence increases
(even if for a short while)

However, these words and my confidence were seen by others
And thereby have become meaningful to them, too.
Now, they share my good fortune.

Published by Loka Hatha Yoga
in Grand Junction, Colorado

There are many suitable places for your meditation.
We hope this becomes one of them.
Anguttara Nikaya 1.159

LOKAHATHAYOGA@GMAIL.COM
(970) 778-2835
lokahathayoga.blogspot.com

Table of Contents

Introduction

This easy to read, English language book was developed to accompany a class series of the same title. However, it has broader applicability, and is useful even to those who were unable to attend, not only for study and practice, but as a model for others to provide similar instruction.

With the intent to permit students to improve personal and professional practice, students are prepared for advanced practice: beginning with introductory background information, skills and conceptual orientation, intermediate classes in training build a foundation of competent practice suitable for advanced classes.

This book presents supporting course material in chronological order, together with other helpful information..

The class was instructed by aaron brachfeld, of the Ashram of Loka Hatha Yoga. aaron was the founding teacher of the Mesa County Jail Yoga program, has served as the Vice Chair of the Grand Valley Interfaith Network where he facilitated the Theological And Knowledge Exchange and has involved himself with numerous other projects besides these, serving a variety of Dharmic and other religious institutions and organizations in various degrees of anonymity, in Grand Junction, Castle Rock, and elsewhere. He says, selfless action is karma yoga.

Initiation

He begins each class by assuring his students he is the worst teacher in the world: they already know everything that he would instruct them in. However, he is there to encourage them in their practice: confidence is the result of extensive practice, and is frequently all that is lacking to begin that performance practice is prepared for. There is no perfection in yoga, but there is sufficiency, and he encourages his students they are good enough to at least begin. In beginning, they will continue their learning by discovering how they are not yet ready, where they need to strengthen better, and then improving, succeed better than if they had by discouragement remained inert in continual training. By such self-education, they achieve the goals of their teachers.

Courage in failure! Failure is the easiest way to see Laxmi, and it is by failure we honor Her. Failure is both the lesson and the means of learning. Sacrifice your failures and gain honor: make each error worthwhile: the price paid for failure (or any tutor) is high, but the knowledge is worth the expense.

The first lesson of his classes is how to recover strength by Asana. This permits students to exert themselves. The second lesson is for the students to learn to not harm themselves. The third lesson is that they exert themselves in practice enough to grow strong enough to do what is necessary. The fourth is to not hesitate in doing all that is necessary, if they are otherwise able and there is opportunity.

He says it is easy to get lazy in each Asana, but the Yogi learns to bear into each pose with all their strength, with all their heart. This is how the Yogi grows their heart stronger!

The Priest in performing the sacrifice for the devotee keeps no honor for themselves, and the devotee, not having performed the sacrifice themselves earns no honor at all. Yet there is honor in sacrifice, and each has done their duty. Through no effort, no action at all, all is accomplished. This is the secret knowledge of sacrifice: it is by this knowledge the purpose of sacrifice is achieved, by which all sacrifices may themselves be sacrificed, and the product of our effort properly enjoyed.

What you will do after this class will seem effortless, and devoid of honor. This speaks to the accomplishment of your teacher, and gives you reason to trust him. Have confidence: he has taken nothing of the honor that was yours, he has taught you nothing you did not know, he has encouraged you to endure, to exert, to achieve that success which you already have earned. And by this successfully taught you to now perform in the exact same way for others.

Everything a teacher should do for their students he has done. You know what you must do now. Having learned from him and his example, do not neglect practice and training. Having practiced and trained sufficiently, succeed - and exceed - him.

Invocation

Om. Om. Om. Sri Ganesh!

Atharva Veda 5, 20

The lion roars for joy during the chase
   expecting the food
The bull bellows for joy battling the yearling
   expecting the heifer
So does the drum whet the voice of the hero
   entering the battle expecting to win

Even when the rules are known and advantage enjoyed
   victory is uncertain
   but loss is yet unreasonable to expect
Having played well, prepare now to gather your winnings
As a gambler holding a high hand
As a Priest preparing for what must be sacrificed
Declare your message pleasantly and clearly:
   it will resound in all directions like thunder
Your voice is counsel and strength to your friends
Songmaker! Give us a song of victory to sing!
Winner - or loser - you will gain honor in this fight
Like a drum, you inspire heroes to success
Even if beaten to pieces!

So now call forth your heroes
And with your friends gathered
Lead us all to honor!

Week 1 and 2

SUMMARY.

Beginner's Class: Introduction to Asanas. Introduction to sacrifice. Introduction to Agni and Svaha. Ganesh. Intermediate Class: Avataras and cosmology.

Training methods

- Use asanas for observing dharma. Recommended asanas: snake, shoulder stand, moon, rabbit, garuda, warrior, and numerous other poses to help student discover dharmic poses (what is easy, sitting comfortably, and what is difficult, sitting with difficulty) with the goal of understanding
    - Ease
    - Difficulty
    - Sufficiency ("middle way")
    - Duty (different than "middle way"): necessity and expedience
    - Endurance required to perform duty
- Use asanas for observing chakras through jnana yoga. Recommended asanas: the dharmic pose (comfortable, difficult), lotus (eyes forward, back straight), king of the fish, mountain (variation, mountain-in-handcuff: self-restraint).
- Use sacrifice to obtain success

Introduction to asanas and sacrifice

Yoga is a practice of uniting body and mind, to strengthen both. It's performed through Asanas, a word which means "rests." Just as sitting is a rest from standing, so is standing a rest from sitting; stillness rests from movement, movement from stillness. Go to Temple and come home; go home and go to work, go to work and then go play. There are millions of Asanas, and it is both impossible to practice them all, and ill advised to. Not all are suitable to your practice.

Hold not long enough, and you won't benefit. Hold too long, and you'll harm yourself – this you shouldn't do. How long to hold an Asana? Svaha! Sufficient, enough, success – this is the secret knowledge by which Yoga is learned.

What is duty? What is Dharma?

Yogi, some Asanas are easier than others, some work is easier than others. Discover your Dharma, your nature, your duty. Knowing your duty, you'll be more ready and rested to do what is difficult and necessary, your Dharma, your nature. Sacrificing for this necessary work becomes easier, as any Asana does. Dharma permits work, Artha, - by tirelessly working the Yogi learns that the benefits of this difficult work, Artha, must be enjoyed, Kama.

A teenager attends to every strand of hair in a mirror before leaving the house: so should you exert self-control. Develop insight for the purpose of self-improvement. Body and mind: it is by self-control one becomes a better person. Yoga is the literal "yoke" for this work. Yogi, learn self-control! Hold the reins and bear the yoke. Perfect your wisdom into contentment.

By Yoga one learns to give up, share, use up, exhaust. This is sacrifice, Yogi! A book has a back cover: put it down when done. Flex, and feel confidence in your strength. Your hard work awaits: seek success, and you will not fail.

What is secret knowledge?

Swami Swatmarama says some things should not be spoken of, and kept secret. The bow lies there for whoever can bend it. The secret lies behind the door: the door is not locked; grow strong enough to open it - and then you will be ready to see what lies on the other side. Then you will be ready for the secret knowledge.

Method for success

It is alright not to know the solution to a problem at the beginning: by study and experimentation, the mechanics are understood, and the causes discerned. Then, several solutions will be apparent. Choosing the best solution means sacrificing objectives to limitations of opportunity and ability: this sometimes means doing nothing at all, to not make things worse. But this is rarely the best course of action. Study the matter, discuss the matter, consult with experts, examine your ability so as to improve your options - then consider what opportunities you have. You will not fail.

The weightlifter does not begin lifting a thousand pounds, nor do they begin by lifting a hundred pounds. They do not begin by lifting a single pound. They begin by learning the skills required for lifting weights safely: they become increasingly flexible and strong by mastering technique through practice.

This is a practice of technique, the gradual strengthening and flexibility which permits a weightlifter to lift first a pound, then a hundred pounds, then a thousand pounds. The practice is not lifting a thousand pounds, that is not success: the athlete is an expert in gaining strength. Strengthen your body and mind.

It seems ironic at first that the training appears to be practices aimed at mastering basic activities, such as sitting, standing, talking, eating, even hygienic self-care. Yet when these are attempted, it is understood that such basic activities actually require considerable strength of body and mind. Such strength is not itself a goal. It permits the understanding, the enlightenment, necessary if we are to bring an end to our suffering.

It is not necessary to understand the mechanics of an automobile to have a smooth ride ("Dukkha," suffering, is a word that connotes a "bad axle hole," a rough ride). If we are suffering from a rough ride, we should grow stronger: it is not practical to repair every road before we travel on it.

A wheel need not be entirely perfectly round to provide a smooth ride: some roads are rougher, and it won't matter whether the wheel is well balanced. The measure of good conscience may be made only after discovering the extent to which the demands of morality are flexible.

We study and practice Yoga to have a smoother ride through Samsara, those cycles of Karma. By understanding the results of our actions, and having the self-control and strength to control our actions, we may achieve better results. You must learn when you must be more flexible - and when you should not, for bending in certain ways will cause as much injury and discomfort as not bending. Every moment of your life is an opportunity to learn when to be flexible, and when to be inflexible. Having begun the path of Hatha Yoga, you will become strong enough to follow it to its end!

Asanas are not acrobatics

Asana is a word that means "sitting." It is similar in many respects to the English "sit," or the romanized "sedes." Sitting is complex, conceptually: a seat is not only something which holds the buttocks, but is an action ("to sit"). But a seat can also be a position of power, or a place (the "seat of power"), it can be a person ("s/he is the Chair of the committee"), it can be a place ("it sits there"). It is a time ("let it sit"). Time, place, action, person.

Asanas are the means of accomplishing the duties: it is not enough that the yoke is borne, the work must be done. Sana means the presentation, or offering, the gain or acquisition of effort: when an A-sana is done, there is nothing left to gain or acquire, there is nothing to present or offer; one has reached, one has accomplished. Like an arrow discharged, there is nothing left for the archer to do: so it is, that when an Asana is performed, there is nothing left for the Yogi to do. One can sit down.

Anyone can become an acrobat, but it is different to become a Yogi. Sit at your desk at work, sit on the bus, sit in your car in traffic. Sit at the dinner table, and sit on the toilet. Sit on the curbside with your neighbor, sit on the battlefield in victory. Your arrow will hit the mark.

The four jnanas

Develop awareness of the body. Watch as you hold an arm still. Watch yourself in any asana. Breathe, counting heartbeats - to better hear your heart: 1 heartbeat, 2 heartbeats, breathe in and hold for 10 heart beats. Sense every fluid in your body, all the air, every muscle, every tendon, the hair touching your clothes, every bone. Smell your nose, taste your mouth, see your eye, hear your ears, feel your skin. Use your body to sense your body. Body is the first jnana.

The sensation is observed through mind: what is smelled, tasted, seen, heard, felt is understood through past experience and the anticipation of future experience, in the context of self and not-self, and other such association. Such bias teaches against trusting sensation, or observation. There is much which is not sensed, or which is ignored. Use your mind to observe your mind. Mind is the second jnana.

This observation is evaluated through consciousness, through complex emotional processes. The act of remembrance, the act of anticipation, all those numerous acts of observation and association produces thought, chemical reactions in the brain which are understood as emotion. Thought, as the basis of all such consideration, may also be considered and evaluated: good and bad, liked and disliked, pleasant and painful. Consideration results in instinctive responses. Some sensations are sought, others avoided. Think about thought. Thought is the third jnana.

This thought is understood in the context of self, identity, soul. I like this, I dislike this, this is Mine, this is not Mine, this is what I am, this is not what I am. Attachment results, desire results, ignorance results, aggression results. But understanding can itself be understood. Understanding is the fourth jnana.

Understanding understanding, understanding the nature of body, mind, thought and self, these can be controlled. This is the foundation of wisdom, of enlightenment, of Bodhi. For it is by effort in self-control that the skill is perfected into numerous siddhis. And by siddhi that contentment (riddhi) is obtained through self-sacrifice.

Jnana (jhana) is a state of rest. It is an asana. It is the means by which increasing awareness is achieved. As you would wake yourself from sleep, rouse yourself from this rest. "Rest" merely implies an inertial resistance: when you are asleep, you tend to stay asleep; when you are awake, you tend to stay awake. Withdraw from sleep, and you wake.

In the first jhana, withdraw from sensuality (touch, taste, sound, sight, smell, etc.): this heightens your ability to think in evaluation.

In the second jhana, withdrawal from thinking in evaluation: this heightens your ability to understand awareness and consciousness.

In the third jhana, where there is awareness of pleasure and pain, freedom of thought and evaluation, freedom of sensuality, you are able to withdraw from elation and distress.

In the fourth jhana you may then withdrawal from seeking pleasure and avoiding pain, or any instinctual response: you may become self-controlled and rational.

In the fourth jhana, direct your mind to withdraw from time, space, form: an increased consciousness and logicality naturally arises. This increased consciousness is necessary for true love: love arises by a knowledge of the nature of things. By merely understanding the basic laws of the universe, freedom from the cycles of suffering is possible. At this stage, there is only wakefulness to truth, and then enlightenment.

Dharma

Do you know your duty? What is duty? What is Dharma? Practicing Asanas, one discovers what is easier, one discovers one's Dharma. What is easy is not right, or wrong. But it is useful to know what is easy if we would accomplish what is difficult. What is difficult is not right, or wrong. But being able to do what is difficult permits us the freedom to accomplish our duty, our Dharma, whether easy or difficult.

Swami Vivekananda describes a duty as an act or work which bears no Karma - good or bad - and thus can help slow the cycle of suffering, and lead to freedom from Samsara. This is the "Karma Yoga," the Yoga by which we control our destiny: whoever controls the effects of their actions is master of their destiny.

Stick your finger in a glass of water and then pull it out: after a moment it will drip and dry; can you see where it was in the water, or even that the water was disturbed? This is your life's work. Though a person may accumulate many things in a lifetime, what they keep when they die is truly theirs. Duties are those actions which are done selflessly, without reward or punishment, fear or desire, without permanence, for their own sake. It is unmotivated and unpurposed - and both voluntarily and consciously undertaken, sometimes with difficulty, sometimes with ease. But always with logical necessity.

Two fools - Angutarra Nikaya 2.98

Who takes upon himself a burden that has not fallen to him is a fool. As is the one who doesn't take up a burden that has fallen to him.

Sacrifice of non-desire, tameness: Nivana

Nivana is non-desire, gaining humanity by non-wildness (tameness, domestication), and is tantamount to freedom from distress: it is the result of perfecting wisdom into contentment. Sacrificing Nivana is the taking up of desire, losing humanity through wildering, letting go of domestication, taking on distress, is sometimes done by conscious purpose and effort (too frequently, it happens unintentionally). Such a sacrifice can only be purposed and selfless when compassion is mastered, and is undertaken to perfect the compassion into love.

Who doesn't want to retire early, and quit work early, to go home - to find moksha in Sannyasa? But though you might live in the Vana, the Forest, and dwell as a Vanaprastha, the desire, the Vana, must be sacrificed to achieve non-desire (ni-vana): first, accomplish Grihastha.

Sannyasa requires the ni-vana sacrifice of Vana-prastha, and this sacrifice requires an altar, which is constructed through the study of architecture, home-making, temple-making, in Grihastha. Such construction cannot be undertaken without study, the seeking of Brahma, the spirit of Agni-Svaha, and all living beings, seen and unseen.

What is placed upon the fire must first be held in hand, and in heart. One must first adopt the worship of the Gods before giving it up, or else it is a practice of atheism, rather than Vedasamnyasa, and Sattrayana. One must make one's self worthy of the self-sacrifice, or else the giving up is defeat and will never know success.

Stories for understanding: Ganesh

The Marriage of Ganesh

Ganesh and His brother Karthikeya shared the same mother and father. But because their mother was in the form of a goddess when she gave birth to Karthikeya, Karthikeya was a deva - whereas Ganesh, being a manifestation of the devoted love between Shiva and Gauri, was not. And with the addition of an elephant's head? What was Ganesh?

Both brothers commanded a great army: Karthikeya commanded the army of devas; Ganesh commanded the Ganas. However, Karthikeya began to think he was superior because he was a Deva - this was not his reasoning, but by nature of his form as a Deva, He was naturally prideful. The two were always bickering, and so one day Shiva proposed they hold a sporting contest to determine who was superior and settle things once and for all.

Both Ganesh and Karthikeya recalled how Shiva had challenged his own brothers to a race to the ends of the universe when they had a similar dispute: Shiva had burned a pillar of light across all space and time, and challenged Brahma and Vishnu to find the end of it. But by the nature of space and time, the pillar bent back around on itself - and both brothers ended up meeting each other in friendship. Shiva said, "this race will be different." Shiva told Karthikeya and Ganesh, "whoever can first circle the entirety of space and time as I did will win the race - and Riddhi, Contentment, the fruit of perfect wisdom."

Karthikeya mounted on his peacock (Karthikeya rode a giant peacock, as a human might ride a horse) and was off. Ganesh's mount was a normal-sized mouse - and at first Ganesh felt quite disadvantaged, as a mouse is slower than a peacock. While his brother rushed off, Ganesh sat down and carefully considered things. He realized his father would not have given him an impossible task. This caused Ganesh to love his father very much, and so Ganesh sought to make Himself worthy of His father's love.

So he devoted Himself to the yoga Shiva had taught him and perfected Wisdom. This act of devotion manifested Buddhi, Knowledge of Wisdom, the beautiful wife of Ganesh. Ganesh then wholly devoted himself to Buddhi, and merging with her, manifested Siddhi, the perfected application of wisdom, his second Wife. Buddhi Ganesh loved Siddhi very much, and she loved Buddhi Ganesh, in turn.

Buddhi Ganesh returned to where Shiva and Gauri waited. Shiva saw the change in Ganesh and smiled benignly, "I see you have found two wives already and do not even ride your vehicle - have you given up?" "No," said Ganesh as he slowly, deliberately, walked around His father and mother, again and again and again, followed closely by Siddhi, and his mouse. "You exist in all of space and time, you are all of space and time. You are my whole universe. I am the manifestation of your love, and I love you." Shiva and Gauri awarded Buddhi Ganesh the victory. "Ganesh, there was no need for you to circle me, you have already won the fruit of Wisdom!"

When Karthikeya returned, he also clearly perceived Buddhi Ganesh's victory, and the way it was won, Karthikeya acknowledged Buddhi Ganesh as the victor, and like a good sport celebrated in the happy marriages of Ganesh. The two brothers were always thereafter reconciled.

Kroncha the Mouse

Kroncha is the vehicle of Ganesh. Kroncha was a clumsy God, who was always accidentally bumping into others, and stepping on toes. Kroncha was also very impolite - not because he didn't want to be, but the wrong words always came out. One day, he stepped on the toes and insulted a powerful sage, who caused him to become a mouse, so that if he ever bumped into someone or stepped on their toes again, he'd at least not cause them any harm or insult – he'd be so small and quiet it wouldn't matter if he was clumsy or rude.

Ganesh is not clumsy, but is not delicate, either. In the end, what is the difference between a lack of delicacy and lack of skill? Intention, care, effort. Ganesh breaks down all obstacles in his way without a care, and needed just such a vehicle as Kroncha: Kroncha's intention, care and effort helps Ganesh's indelicacy at least not cause harm.

When Ganesh met Kroncha (now a mouse), it was because Kroncha accidentally bumped into Ganesh and stepped on his toes, then rudely addressed Ganesh. Ganesh understood the potential for Kroncha immediately, and Kroncha saw his ability to be useful. The two hit it off and became good friends, despite their total lack of social charm, mutually insulting each other and bruising each other. It was only natural Ganesh would take out his lasso and throw it around Kroncha's neck to leap on – and has ridden Kroncha as a vehicle ever since (Kroncha has carried Ganesh ever since).

The Birth of Ganesh

Ganesha is the manifestation of Gauri's love for Shiva.

Gauri manifested Her love for Shiva in the form of a child while Shiva was out of the house, performing profound devotions to Gauri. It was the day after Gauri was herself manifested, and had come home to Shiva's house. After manifesting Ganesh, Gauri took a ritual bath - and asked Ganesh to protect her while performing this ritual bath.

Shiva returned home during this bath to discover a small child standing at the entrance of his house, denying him entrance. He did not recognize the child, nor did he see it was the reflection of Gauri's love for him. Shiva asked the squadron of Ganas standing guard at the entrance who the child was, and whether anyone had been permitted into the house while he was gone? The Ganas said they had guarded the house, but they did not know who the child was. Shiva commanded the Ganas to open his house for him - but the small child easily withstood them. Shiva then summoned all his armies of Ganas, but Ganesh withstood them all. Shiva called upon all his devotees, and they all were destroyed by this small child. Shiva called upon Brahma, and Vishnu, to help - but they too were defeated. Shiva grew angry, and himself approached Ganesh - and after a protracted battle, struck off Ganesh's head - but only after Ganesh recognized Shiva as his father, and happily lay down before Shiva, and submitted to the blow.

It was at this moment that Gauri heard a disturbance outside, and came to see Ganesh killed. Gauri was enraged at the disrespect Shiva had paid to her devotion, and manifesting as a very wrathful Shakti, explained the situation to a terrified Shiva: Shakti threatened to destroy the world if Ganesh were not restored to life. But poor Ganesh's head had been destroyed. Brahma suggested Ganesh might recover if given a new head. The suggestion seemed absurd, and likely only to irritate Shakti further. Shiva did not know what to do!

Shakti took pity on Shiva, and resumed her form as Gauri. Gauri ordered the Ganas to search the world and bring Her the head of any creature that was sleeping with its head facing north. The entire world was searched in an instant: only one creature was at that moment sleeping in that position. It was an elephant, belonging to Indra, the King of the Gods [who has his own stories, which end here: Indra has no more need of a vehicle after this]. The elephant woke, and understanding the situation, permitted the Ganas to take his head, sacrificing it to Shiva-Gauri. The elephant then put itself peacefully back to sleep, and while the elephant slept, the squadron of Ganas cut off its head and brought instantly before Gauri and Shiva. Shiva attached the head of the elephant to Ganesh's neck.

Understanding the nature of the devotion Ganesh represented, and the insight Ganesh held in recognizing Shiva even when Shiva did not recognize Ganesh, Shiva instructed every being to seek Ganesh before undertaking any significant undertaking, for Ganesh had already proven He was Master of all obstacles. Even after Ganesh fell, Shiva was unable to enter his own house: now he would still not enter, except with Ganesh's permission. Shiva placed Ganesh, His son, in command of the Ganas whom He had conquered.

Ganesh would soon have many adventures, and manifest Buddhi, Siddhi and Riddhi - his three wives. With whom he manifested numerous children, each exemplifying satisfaction.

Not by Moonlight

One practice which is not practiced on Ganesh Chaturthi is moon watching: once, the moon had laughed when Ganesh tripped and fell, and for this Ganesh prohibited His students from learning from the moon(light) upon penalty of being falsely believed to be a criminal yogi, and dishonored. Vishnu, a student of Ganesh, once broke this prohibition - and has ever since in every manifestation been falsely accused, believed to be criminal: for example, Krishna was falsely accused of theft, the Buddha was accused of teaching atheism, Rama was expelled on false accusations.

However, if the moon is accidentally meditated on or studied, relieve the penalty by performing difficult asanas: perfect your practice of Ganesh's yoga during Ganesh Chaturthi.

Shiva Maha-Purana 2.109 - Many Ganeshes

The endless repetitions present in the stories demonstrate the generalities and exceptionalities particular to any rendition: in life, too, there are generalities and exceptionalities, and it is an expression of statistical science to learn from what is exceptional only in context to what is general in understanding the reason why things have turned out differently than expected.

One of the literary forms of Hinduism is this form of variable repetition: much as a sketch artist will use multiple lines on paper to show general forms, and fewer lines to show definite forms. Or in the way that a journey (yatra) is undertaken many times, each time the trail is somewhat different as seasons change, as weather changes, as other travelers are passed. This literary form also helps a reader learn the information presented. However, though this literary form is often tedious in its plodding redundancy, it builds a strength of patience and attention to detail.

A small taste is presented here by telling a variant of the above stories: the avoidance of moonlight, the practice of jnana yoga, the manifestation of Ganesh and Kroncha, etc.

Brahma said, there have been many various Ganeshas in the many Kalpas. During the Shweta Kalpa, Ganesh was born to Shiva and Parvati, when they went to Kailash Mountain shortly after their marriage.

Parvati had decided to take a bath, and instructed Nandi to let no one enter the home without her permission. During her bath, Shiva arrived by chance. Despite Nandi faithfully conveying the message, Shiva went inside anyway - for it was his home, after all. Parvati did not like this at all - for it was also her home. She realized Nandi could not actually prevent Shiva from entering, so before her next bath she took the dirt from her body and made Ganesha. She instructed Ganesha to not allow anyone in without her permission - and gave him a stick as a weapon. By chance again, Shiva again arrived during the bath - he tried to ignore Ganesha but Ganesha was able to block the door.

Shiva realized at once that Ganesh could not be his servant - for if he was, like Nandi, he could not actually prevent him from entering his own home. At the same time, he was frustrated and furious. Shiva ordered the Ganas which accompanied him to kill Ganesh - Shiva rarely went anywhere without his Ganas (perhaps you can see why Parvati would want privacy during her bath?)

The Ganas attacked Ganesha, but none were a match for him. After being defeated by Ganesha, the Ganas went to Shiva, and asked what to do? At that moment, Brahma and Vishnu, together with many Gods, noticing Shiva was home, came to visit (perhaps you can see why Parvati would want privacy during her bath?)

Brahma decided he would reason with Ganesh. But as soon as he got close enough to Ganesh, Ganesh attacked Brahma! Shiva rushed to defend his brother, and then fought Ganesha in single combat. At first, Ganesh dominated the battle, and was at the point of overcoming Shiva. Shiva realized at that moment that he could show no restraint with Ganesh - and so, with his full strength, he utterly destroyed the head of Ganesha with his Trident.

Parvati had been admiring Ganesha, and saw his death. At the death of her valiant servant, she grew so angry that she manifested every one of the forms of Shakti, and began to destroy every world. The devas were terrified, and sought the protection of Shiva, Brahma and Vishnu - but found no refuge. So the devas begged Shakti for mercy. Shakti said the condition of her pardon would be that Ganesha would be brought back to life - and equal to any of the devas, equal to even Shiva, Vishnu, or Brahma.

The devas begged Shiva to make Ganesha alive again. Shiva perceived the danger clearly, and knew there was no shame in being overmatched by Shakti's strength. But Ganesh's head had been completely destroyed! So he and sought about for a new head - and asked his brothers, and all the devas to help him. Some offered them their own heads - but not any head would do - they would need to go north of there, and find and a head facing north. Indra commanded his vehicle, an elephant, to lay down and face north - at the same time that the Goddess Malini, drinking the the bath water of Parvati (which contained those bits of dirt that she had not removed to make Ganesh), gave birth to Parvati's desire - a reincarnated Ganesh. But this reincarnation had 5 elephant heads (because Malini had birthed him). Shiva combined the dead body with the reincarnation and the head of Indra's elephant. To confirm that Ganesh was in fact equal to anyone, all the devas worshiped him in the way they would worship Brahma, Vishnu, Shiva or Shakti - and Brahma, Vishnu and Shiva all acknowledged him as their equal. Shakti was pacified, and retook the form of Parvati.

Ganesha had an "older" brother, Kartikeya. The two got along well, except once. Both wanted to be married first - Kartikeya said, he was eldest. But Ganesh said he was equal to Shiva, Brahma, Vishnu - and any God, and deserved the honor by right. Shiva and Parvati consulted together to find a solution to this problem: they told their two sons that whoever would return first after circumambulating every world would get married first.

Ganesh thought he was at a disadvantage, as Kartikeya's vehicle was a peacock and could fly very fast - much faster than Ganesh's mouse. After setting out, Ganesh received some help - Vishnu and Brahma helped him understand! And he found a wife, Buddhi, who also helped him become so much smarter. So Ganesh returned to his parents and asked them to sit together. He circumambulated them and said, "according to the Veda, circumambulating one's parents give virtues equivalent to that of circumambulating the whole earth. So, now you must get me married first." Shiva and Parvati were both very impressed by his intelligence. So they arranged for him to be married to Siddhi and Riddhi, the daughters of Vishwaroop Prajapati. In due course of time, they had two sons: Kshem and Labh.

Eventually Kartikeya returned from his journey, and saw Ganesh had already been married - and had sons. He felt sad, as if he had been cheated. And began to feel jealous. He greeted his whole family, then went off to Kraunch Mountain to meditate. Parvati felt the sadness of her son, and so she and Shiva went on pilgrimage to Kraunch Mountain. This is why having a Darshan of Kartikeya (studying Kartikeya) on the full moon day of Kritika Nakashatra is so auspicious, for remembering how Shiva and Parvati comforted Kartikeya destroys the regrets of lack of intelligence or strength.

[Kartikeya eventually married Devasena and Valli, and lived happily ever after, too - with Ganesh, Siddhi, Riddhi, Kshem, and Labh - but that is another story]

Artharva Veda 6, 71

Whatever food I eat, whatever I require to sustain me, whether gold, or bloody meat, I hope it was sacrificed and obtained rightly, and that I am worthy of it. Whether sacrificed and obtained rightly or not, whether or not I am worthy, I sacrifice my doubt, unburden myself of doubt. I am in need of sustenance now. I must hope it is wholesome. Even poison may taste sweet, so now I hope that what sustenance I take and swallow if poisonous, or unwholesome, is at least sweet. I have reason to hope, and hold confidence, for even Agni accepts and eats all which is presented, whether sacrificed rightly or wrongly, obtained rightly or wrongly, provided willingly or unwillingly. Even if it extinguishes the flame. I will become like Agni.

Week 3 and 4

SUMMARY

Beginner's Class: Introduction to Jnana Yoga. Introduction to Chakras. Introduction to Bhakti Yoga. Intermediate Class: Ahimsa and the sacrifice of food. Sacrifice of Ahimsa. Mind reading. Gauri. Annapurna.

Training methods

- Technical training in jnana yoga skills, including
    - Asanas. Recommended asanas: sitting comfortably, sitting with difficulty, lotus, corpse, parusha, mountain.
    - Preparation for jnana yoga: Hatha Yoga
    - Directed meditation
    - Undirected meditation
    - Mastering instinct
    - Awareness
    - Self-improvement through Bhakti Yoga
- Technical training in the food sacrifice
    - Ahimsa
    - Annapurna
    - Sat-sangha (satsang)

Preparing for Jnana Yoga by Hatha Yoga: Instruction in Indra puja

Preparations for Jnana Yoga are the same for which would be undertaken for any considerable exertion. Besides strength and endurance training (mental, sensory, physical, etc.) the yogi will benefit from flexing their strength before beginning, to make mind and body more pliable.

The nose is cleaned of mucus, as is the chest. The bowels are emptied of fecal matter, the bladder emptied of urine, the skin is washed, the eyes are cleaned of dust and tears, the ears cleaned of wax, the hair shortened or tidied - and more is done besides this to permit the body's readiness, according to the particular form of the body of the Yogi. Attention to form!

The sacrifice of these fluids is puja, the giving up of what is attached to, seen as self, for the purpose of honoring the purpose of the yogi for which they are given up. And for this, attachment to form is made: what is laid down must be first taken up.

Appropriate clothing is worn, sufficient nutrient and water consumed, and other items accepted which will be necessary to the work: the sacrifice of these items to the yogi is the same puja, honoring the purpose of the yogi who would use them. The room and world itself is prepared for the exertion: this preparation is also the same puja, honoring the purpose of the yogi. These are the essential expressions of Indra Puja.

The Yogi will exhaust themselves, and by preparing for that moment beyond total exertion when strength is recovered, and expended again, anticipating failure to be followed by success honors Indra, the second wind. The athlete prepares for themselves a drink of cold water, the storekeeper covers for their employee during lunch break: there is trust that what is lost will return.

Prior to beginning yoga, prior to igniting the sacrificial fire, the Yogi confirms their intent and ability to persist until strength returns, and their secret knowledge that strength, if exhausted, must return.

Then, the yogi is ready to feed the sacrificial fire: and Agni, the sacrificial fire, whether the heat of a flame, or the bodily heat of exertion, the light of the mind's awareness, the burning love felt by self, must be fed. The abhishekam is not performed by milk or water or precious herbs - but by Hatha yoga.

Hatha yoga is the process by which the world, body and mind is "forced" - whether difficult or easy, Jnana is not something which naturally occurs. Hatha is the process by which success is "struck" (as in striking gold, or striking a blow in battle: here the yogi battles their body, mind, thought and self, for self-improvement).

The exertion toward self-improvement will necessitate breaks for recovering strength: these asanas, these rests, achieve the purpose of the practice as much as the self-improvement which is undertaken during the exertion.

Strength recovered, strength expended, strength built slowly, the athlete eventually perceives a duty to exert their strength: this achieves the purpose of Jnana yoga.

Sitting in Jnana, the yogi feels their breath leave, and return, the pause between heartbeats, and is increasingly aware of death and ending, the return of life. This is how the Yogi understands that ignorance, sleep, even death, is merely a form of rest, merely another asana - one which utterly destroys the yogi, but one which nevertheless is recovered from.

Technical training in practice

The Buddha Gotama said that a person may practice for their own benefit, for the benefit of others, for both the benefit of themselves and others, or neither for their own benefit nor for that of others. However, regardless of the initial reasons for practice, a person comes by degrees to practice for the benefit of themselves and others. Just as milk naturally separates into cream if left alone, just as butter naturally arises from churning milk, the best of a person's nature naturally arises through practice - whether that practice is undertaken selfishly and alone or for the betterment of others with others.

As a fighter will inevitably lose after too many battles, so too will the yogi eventually be overcome by themselves when they fight constantly against their nature: the yogi will inevitably succeed.

Observe your enemy, yourself. Understand the cycle of emotions, the cycle of thoughts, learn to anticipate yourself, your thought, your mind, your body. This is undirected meditation. Training in undirected meditation provides sufficient strength to achieve each asana of jnana yoga.

Using body against body, mind against mind, thought against thought, self against self, by Hatha, as you would train an animal, or a child, or a loyal employee, train yourself. Build new habits, build a new nature. Obtain new skills and develop them. This, and other similar work, is directed meditation. Training in directed meditation provides sufficient strength to achieve each asana of jnana yoga.

You will discover instinct, the limitations of your form. You are human. Emotional, thoughtful, perceptive, imaginative, desiring, aggressive, ignorant. There are so many instincts. Master them. To be afraid of the dark does not require one cower inside until dawn. Be afraid of the dark, love yourself for your humanity, but also perform your duty. Then you can become something more than human.

Aware of yourself, aware of what is more than self, aware of other selves, aware of what is greater than human, manifest these greater forms. As a person would merge with a horse as a vehicle, or gain the spatial awareness of their truck, or freely express themselves with a pen or phone, merge with your tools, your vehicles. Then manifest new forms, to use new tools, new vehicles. Observe your previous and future manifestations, and the manifestations of others, discover the secret knowledge of avatara.

Having used Hatha Yoga to train in Jnana Yoga, having trained in Jnana Yoga, you will be prepared to practice Bhakti Yoga.

Practice Jnana - Anguttara Nikaya 5.73

One of the monks there went to the Buddha Gotama, and asked, "you talk about 'dwelling in Dharma,' please explain and expound on this?"

The Buddha said,

A monk might study the Dharma, spending the day in study. This monk is keen on studying the Dharma, but does not dwell in the Dharma.

A monk might take the Dharma as he has heard it - faithfully! - and teaches it in full detail to another. He spends the day describing the Dharma. This monk is keen on describing the Dharma, but does not dwell in the Dharma.

A monk might recite the Dharma, and be keen on reciting the Dharma - but does not dwell in the Dharma.

A monk might think about the Dharma, evaluating it, examining it, keen on thinking - but not dwelling in the Dharma.

But there is a monk who, having studied, described it, thought upon it, lives according to what he has studied, described and thought upon. He dwells in the Dharma. But, understanding this is still not sufficient - it is not sufficient to dwell in the Dharma, monk.

Practice jnana, monk.

Whatever a teacher should do I have already done for you. You know what you must do. Exert yourself now: practice jnana, monk. Over there are roots of trees suitable for this, over there are empty dwellings also suitable for this.

Alone, eyes open or closed

It is neither necessary nor useful to practice alone, or in the company of others. Whether you have been trained to practice eyes open or eyes closed, perception is still the same. It is good to train both eyes open and eyes closed, if only to understand this similarity.

When Yoga, whether Hatha, or Jnana, or Karma, or Bhakti, or any other form of Yoga, becomes established, Pranayama is possible. The best understanding of Pranayama is the pause between study and practice. It is the moment when breath stops - when love so fills the body, mind and heart that our breath is taken away - the moment of redeath, and rebirth.

Yoga is practiced so that upon success, the practice may be stopped.

Swami Sivananda said that such a moment permits us to perceive within ourselves numerous faults: for we finally understand what our goal is.

More importantly, it is then that we notice the limitations of Yoga. Then, like a smith burning, beating and blowing away the impurities of gold, we turn our strength inwards. And begin to breathe again.

Take your very first first breath!

Swami Swatmarama says that merely learning to sit and control the breath is sufficient to the establishment of Yoga, for within that simple act is the knowledge required to master ourselves and eat healthy and moderate food. The practice of Pranayama, this purification, will naturally result.

The Buddha Gotama asked, who, upon passing by a mirror and seeing their face covered in filth, will not try to clean it? Or noticing a stain in their clothing will not wash their clothes?

The Yogi in Pranayama clings to life; they are not ready to die, for they clearly see their work. They will cling to each breath. Indeed, the sensation of redeath and rebirth is such that a breath is naturally inhaled, almost spasmodically. Like being doused in cold water and quickly waking up from a dream! How then the Yogi succeed in their goal, when desiring and attached to life? By purifying themselves, they will unattach, and uncling; the breath becomes more regular. They learn to live - and die - in continence, one breath at a time.

Do you have the strength to await death like a temp worker or day-worker waiting for their pay at the end of the day, performing their duty to the end? Then, to quit when their boss tells them to go home? Can you remain at work as long as required, and no longer?

Once regularity in breath is gained, the Yogi begins to control the manner of their breath: faster, slower, through one side of their nose, than the other; exhaling through alternate nostrils - quite as easily as most of us would eat on one side of the mouth or another. Invigorated, they practice morning, noon, evening, and midnight; four times a day, they practice and rest. Like breathing in and out.

Then, the Yogi begins to flex their strength: their practice becomes constant. Day and night, driven by self-improvement, and without exhaustion or weariness, motivated by love and compassion, they perform the duty of their birth within their Ashrama. They do not suffer from disease, nor do they suffer from discomfort of any kind. They are not motivated by pleasure or praise. They desire only success!

Their duties become more secretive, more anonymous, as they become more natural; praise and pleasure are avoided as much as pain and punishment are not avoided; the action of life becomes as selfless as any act of Yoga!

The duties of a Yogi are merely purification (Dhauti), digestion (Basti), discerning truth through logic (Neti), awareness or perception (Trataka), flexing or exertion every moment of body and heart and mind (Nauti) and passive or non-action (Kapala Bhati). In the four Ashramas, these duties are undertaken in different ways. While some Yogis will actually physically cleanse their nostrils and even their bowels, this is not the appropriate practice for all Ashramas, where discerning truth through logic and expelling what is foul might be best accomplished in matters of business and trade, or in the protection of a community through the establishment of justice.

Living alone - Samyutta Nikaya 35.63

Migajala asked the Buddha Gotama, "you have taught to live alone, but I cannot understand how is this done? Whether a person dwells in a busy village or in the wilderness, it would seem they are never alone."

Gotama said, "though a person may live even in a crowded city, they may live alone – if they leave behind their pursuit of pleasure and avoidance of pain. A person who seeks pleasure or avoids pain is never alone, even in remote forests, far from the noise and business of crowded cities. A person need not persist in their desire for pleasure or avoidance of pain, they need not persist in their attachment to things they have seen, heard, smelled, tasted, touched or thought. A person can indeed live alone, even in a crowded city."

Living with yourself – Samyutta Nikaya 21.10

When the Buddha Gotama was staying near Rajagaha in the Bamboo Grove in the Squirrel's sanctuary, a monk whose name was Thera lived alone and extolled the virtues of living alone, without association, by himself. He begged for alms alone, sat alone in meditation, walked in meditation alone. One day, a large number of monks brought to Gotama's attention how Thera was so alone and so Gotama asked Thera to come to him.

Thera came at once. Gotama asked him if he was, in fact, alone, without association. "Yes, Sir," said Thera. "I am always alone."

Gotama said, "Thera, there is a difference between being alone and being by yourself. Only when you abandon your past, and relinquish your future, and no longer desire, no longer avoid, then you travel with no companion and live perfectly alone, whether you are surrounded by others or not. Otherwise you are by yourself, associating with your past, your future, your desires, your aversions, you are not alone."

Release of urine, mind – Anguttara Nikaya 6.42

Gotama said, when I am traveling along a road and see no one in front or behind me, at that time I have my ease, even when urinating and defecating. You do not always need companions. Fend off gain and fame, and all responsibilities. Dispel drowsiness and fatigue. Do not neglect seclusion, do not neglect isolation. Attend to perception, concentrate your mind, release your mind.

Sacrifice of Ahimsa

It is necessary to give up ahimsa, non-harm, if one is to practice compassion. It is necessary too to give up sympathy to practice compassion.

Consider, when a lion hunts, captures, kills and eats a sheep, it is as wrong for you to feel the pain of the sheep as it is to feel the joy of the lion. Indeed, both views are limited. Sympathy is limited. Did it not occur to you that the lion is defending the plants from the sheep: where is your sympathy for these beings? Some would, out of sympathy, refrain from building a house without harming the earthworms displaced by the foundation - what of all those beings which rely on the grasses and trees displaced by the house? What of their shelter, their home, their food? The lion harms the sheep, it is true, but this blood spilt is a righteous sacrifice. The sheep, without the lions, would cause regrettable harm.

The lion, the sheep, the grass - each are closely related. When it is understood that a human and an earthworm share more than half their genetic material, and descended from a common ancestor, each requiring the same amino acids to survive, each eating of the same vegetable matter, sharing the same home and world, it is possible to understand the common ancestry each shares with the plants they require for food, and the lion which protects these plants from the sheep. It is possible to see the brotherhood shared with worm, lion, sheep and plant, to see the brotherhood shared with all other people. We are all the same expression of life.

And it is possible, upon understanding the generations of your family, stretching through the eons, to the lion, the sheep, the worm, the plant, even the bacteria in your wounds, to understand then the nobility of all living creatures, and the essential importance of every individual. As each type of being has perfected its existence to a way of life, a niche, each individual by the facts of its survival proves that it is good enough for the challenges of its specific duty in this world. You, too, are uniquely suited to a place and time. Do you not yet know your duty?

It is not by birth that one is ennobled, becoming the envy of Indra and Brahma. It is by self-control that one betters oneself. It is by sacrificing this self, by the ritual of self-sacrifice in your Ashrama, that you can achieve the full promise of your humanity - and come to cultivate true compassion, even for sheep.

Sacrifice of Food

The Buddha Gotama taught that compassion for all living creatures was necessary, and recognizing that our food comes from damaging or killing both animal and plant life is important toward understanding the nature of our own suffering. "Be aware of what your food was and is, and how it became so, before eating it" (Mahavagga VI.23.9).

What use is it to prolong our lives another day, or year, when we will eventually die? For what did these beings die? Why did the farmers work in poverty, or enslaved, to sustain you? Why did you defend yourself against microbes and insects and other predators? Why did you defend yourself against your enemies? Are you worthy of these sacrifices - for so many beings have died or been harmed for your sake, to honor your purpose.

Once there was a soybean, and it was planted in the deep rich soil of the river valley. It did not know the river. It did not know that the river came from a distant mountain, having fallen from heaven. It did not know of heaven – or hell. It did not even know its farmer, who took the river and brought it to irrigate the valley, and protected it from its many unknown enemies.

The soybean set down roots, and grew above the soil, connected biochemically through the soil and air with the other soybeans around it, and even with the strange, wild plants that sometimes grew among them. It lived long days, and set fruit, pollinated by bees and beetles, mosquitoes and flies. It was happy until the day it died, content with its children. Its children, embryonic in their mother's womb, could have been planted in the same valley as their mother, but were chosen by their farmer for sale. The farmer did not know what would happen to the soybeans, but loading them on his truck, took them far away from the valley.

By chance – simple chance – the soybeans were sold several times before being owned by a manufacturer, who chose them to make the ink with which you read these words. And one of those beans, by chance – simple chance – having been cared for by the farmer, traded by the merchant, crafted by the manufacturer into ink, now, by my own care, has become the word "enlightened."

Along the way, that bean was protected and fed. Countless beings protected and fed it: microorganisms mineralized nitrogen, cattle provided manure, spiders defended it from its enemies. It was carried and protected and fed by the help of metals found deep within the earth which had been sought for by miners, crafted by blacksmiths, into semiautonomous robots - advanced computers with the rudimentary beginnings of artificial intelligence, little less aware than the bean they help craft. This is so unlikely, such a small chance, that it is a miracle.

The paper, once a tree, was pulped with similar care and it was only chance that the tree would carry that word of enlightenment, bonding with the ink. In that random marriage of soybean and tree, the tree serves the noble purpose of bringing you to greater awareness – as I do. As my computer does, in shaping the ink.

And the cattle that fed the soybean with their manure, the farmer, the merchant, the manufacturer – they were fed by the soybean's minor companions. These soybeans fed, too, the weavers who made the clothing required by the farmers and miners, the manufactuers and computer engineers. And these people were sheltered in houses built from the minor companions of the pulped tree, each having yielded up quality timber for that purpose with their lives.

You may trust the words I caused to be written with the ink on this paper, for they were made not by me alone, but by a Sangha, natural and artificial, all of whom are purposed for the relief of your suffering.

And though it was the purest chance that brought you to read these words, consider the pure chance that brought them to be written: the good fortune of a single soybean, or a tree, to become enlightened may become your own – if you allow yourself to become transformed and shaped, as they were. Ink is easily shaped with patience and care. An animal is easily trained with patience and care. Can you not shape and train yourself? Develop your skill in body, mind and heart.

It is possible to develop your skill. If it were not possible to develop your skill, I would not tell you to develop your skill. If this development of skillfulness was conducive to harm, I would not direct you toward development of your skill. But because this development is to your benefit, I urge you to develop your skill.

Abandon what is unskillful. It is possible to abandon those behaviors of body, mind and heart that are unskillful. If it were not possible to abandon them, I would not tell you to abandon them. But because it is possible to abandon them, I tell you to abandon them. If this abandoning caused you harm, I would not direct you toward that abandoning. But because the abandonment is conducive to what is beneficial, I urge you to abandon what is unskillful.

As you eat your food, listen to this sat-sangha, perceive the web of life which you have spun, and you are caught in: speak with those whom you wander on with. We would encourage you, with one voice: surely, if even a plant can become enlightened, we believe that you can, too.

Anguttara Nikaya 4.77: causes of illogic

The Buddha Gotama said: illogic is caused, among other things, by conjecture upon false premises. He said, any conjecture from these false-premises will result in illogic, in irrationality, madness, insanity, dissatisfaction, vexation and frustration.

(1) Any conjecture on the origin of things, their moment and nature and cause of creation, must begin with a false premise. And any conjecture on the termination of things, their moment and cause of destruction, must

begin with a false premise. This is because all phenomenon and their natures, all Dharma, are emergent properties co-arising from co-dependent conditions, and these are the very conditions which cause their co-termination. With the moment of creation and the moment of destruction occurring simultaneously, and interdependently, it is evident that there is no force, no power inherent within anything: for these are themselves emergent properties.

A wave cannot be caused, except when there is energy and form for it to bring into motion. And because of the resistance of the form to energy, because of the energy's wavelike nature which results in that resistance, the wave co-arises with the cause of its termination. Similarly, fire emerges from fuel, air, and spark - and the nature of these create the conditions for its extinguishment. Life itself, consciousness itself, self, identity, "soul" - these, too, are emergent properties, created at the moment of their destruction, sustained through interdependent factors, with no inherent existence of their own. To one who truly understands, neither "finite" nor "infinite" can describe the universe, for it must exist beyond space; neither "eternal" nor "non-eternal" can apply to what exists beyond time.

(2) Any conjecture on the precise consequences of actions, or things in action, must begin with a false premise. Uncertainty and randomness, chaos, must be accepted as a premise and any consequence can only be anticipated or predicted within degrees of confidence, conditionally, and limitedly. Because of limitations of observation, as well as the interdependent nature of observer and observed, as well as limitations of understanding, and the nature of phenomenon.

(3) Any conjecture on the powers that one may manifest or realize while absorbed in Jnana or other Yoga must begin with a false premise. Power, whether innate or manifested (Avatara), is an emergent property of energy and form, which are also co-arising, co-dependent, co-terminating. There is no inherent power to realize, or manifest. No enlightenment; no buddhi, no siddhi, no riddhi. Nor any other power of a Yogi.

(4) And the Buddha said, so too, must any conjecture on the power

manifested in Me, or in any Buddha (as differs from power manifested by a Buddha), begin with a false premise.

Anguttara Nikaya 10.96: the belief

When Ananda was staying at Rajagaha at the Tapoda monastery, one night he decided to go to the Tapoda hot springs to bathe his limbs.

When morning came and he was drying off from his bath and was dressing to go, Kokanuda, a wanderer, approached the hot springs and, seeing a monk at the springs, Kokanuda asked Ananda what kind of a monk he was?

Ananda said that he was a student of the Buddha Gotama.

Kokanuda asked Ananda if he could clarify some questions about particular lessons of the Buddha Gotama that were very confusing. Ananda promised to answer them, if he knew the answer.

"Do you Buddhists believe that the cosmos is eternal?"

Ananda shook his head, "no, we do not."

"So you think the cosmos is not eternal?"

Ananda again shook his head, "no, we do not."

Kokanuda was confused. "Do you think that the cosmos is finite?"

"No, we do not."

"Then you think the cosmos is infinite?"

"No, we do not."

Kokanuda was again confused.

"Do you think that there is a soul in the body?"

"No, we do not."

"Then you think there is no soul in the body?"

"No, we do not."

"Do you believe you exist after death?"

"No, we do not."

"Then you think that you do not exist after death?"

"No, we do not."

Kokanuda was becoming frustrated. "Do you believe anything?"

"Friend," said Ananda, "it is not the case that we believe, or do not believe. A belief requires an apprehension of truth, and this apprehension would require a valuation of that truth, that one belief is valuable, and another is worthless. Knowledge is a belief, seeing is a belief, hearing is a belief, touching is a belief."

Ananda said, "We believe only that there are beliefs. These beliefs are taken up, held, obsessed upon. We believe that having been taken up, beliefs are then held. Having been held, beliefs are obsessed upon. We believe that the ignorance of truth creates a desire for belief, and this causes a hatred of what is contrary to that belief. We believe that beliefs cause suffering. But we also believe that beliefs can be let go and uprooted."

Anguttara Nikaya 10.51: Mind reading

Gotama was staying at Anathapindika's monastery near Savatthi when he was asked by a monk during an assembly how to become skilled in reading the minds of others.

Gotama said before becoming skilled in reading the minds of others, one should become skilled in reading their own mind.

Even as a young man or young woman would use the reflection of a mirror, or even still water, to clean dirt and blemishes from their face to beautify themselves, so should you examine your mind and remove unskillful qualities from it.

Consider what you desire, if you maintain thoughts of ill will, if you are overcome by drowsiness and laziness, or restlessness, if you are uncertain, angry, if you have thoughts of pleasure and pain, if you are unconcentrated? And why?

These are not necessarily undesirable qualities: just as a person whose head or hat was on fire would become aware of the fire by looking in a mirror and then desire the fire extinguished, and would put forth extra effort and become restless, of single mind after becoming alerted to the fire, in the same way should you become alerted to the unskillful, evil qualities in your mind.

And, just as a person whose head or hat were not on fire would find in a mirror they are beautiful, and then use that mirror for polishing their beauty, you may become alert to the fact that you are skillful; then your duty is to make an effort in maintaining that skill, and using that skill toward ending your suffering for the benefit of all beings.

Stories for practice: Gauri

Uma Aparna

When Shakti took the form of Parvati, she was a Deva: the adopted daughter of a mountain and a being which is best understood by the word "nymph" (an "aspara," the spirit of a cloud or water). She was one of three sisters: Her adopted sisters devoted also themselves to Shiva, and to demonstrate their devotion ate only a single leaf for their food every day. This represented the very minimum required for life (for a creature like they were: the cross-breed of a mountain and a nymph). But Sati knew Her true nature (as a Deva - and as Shakti), and thus she required no food at all - She only required the love of Shiva. She gave up eating entirely, to gain the attention of Shiva and demonstrate Her true nature to him. Her starvation gained the attention of her parents and sisters, too; astonished and overawed, though they had known she was a Deva, they did not really understand it - now they understood her true nature, and even saw she was Shakti, Love itself.

She was first called by them Aparna, one who eats nothing. Then they called her Uma! The name implies a combination of "Oh, mother!" "Oh, beautiful!" (Shakti is a "mother" of all beings, and is "beautiful"), this is an exclamation similar to the English "Oh, don't!" (Parvati's austerity seemed unnecessarily cruel, but in fact was required to gain the attention of Shiva, and preserve Parvati's life). This was an exclamation of beauty, splendor and tranquility - in so many more ways than these, the name represents the moment when her family understood her true nature.

"Uma" is also, however, a masculine term for a wharf or landing place - when it is remembered that Shakti is partially female and partially male, partially Shiva, the concept that She was presenting a landing place for Shiva is also understood better in the context that She was presenting herself to Shiva, not so much as an offering (how could She offer herself, when She was partially Shiva?) but in the sense of permission and availability. As a wharf or landing place may be beautiful enough to entice a traveler, She appeared so beautiful.

"Uma" is the state of being her sisters were attempting to achieve, but which only Parvati might.

Annapurna

Annapurna is a name that means "perfect nutrient" or "perfect food": the eating without hunger or desire, for the pure purpose of nourishment, the nourishment that nourishes and sustains anything and everything.

Shiva once said that because all form is illusion, all things are Maya, the need for nourishment is also illusion. Though food could not be had without Himsa, harm, it would be possible, said Shiva, to not cause harm by simply not eating. Gauri, who was a reflection of Maya, disagreed with Shiva: all food was obtained by Himsa, it was true, but still, everyone had to eat. Not eating was self-harm. That is why it is difficult. But Shiva was not persuaded.

So, to prove her position, Gauri caused all nourishment to disappear: no matter what a being ate, now that food could not be had. Plants, animals, people, even Shiva suffered famine, surrounded by food. Seeing the beings distressed, and that Shiva had learned her lesson, Gauri then produced a magic Kitchen, and fed every being what most nourished them – and in the line for nourishment was Shiva, begging with a bowl. He was humble, and said "I now understand nourishment, whether physical or spiritual, is no illusion. I understand now you are Maya, you are the source of all all food, you are Annapurna." Gauri, now called Annapurna, fed Shiva with her own hands, and instructed him in the Dharma, the duty and nature, of nourishment, and in the necessity for the sacrifice of food. Not being able to refrain from harming another being, we must become worthy of the sacrifice of their lives: food is not merely intended to sustain our existence. And we must nourish others.

The Buddha Gotama instructed that before eating, the origin and necessity of the nourishment should be understood: life is sustained by death, and the sacrifice and gift made by the beings we use for food should be respected by right living – that our strengthening succeeds in preparing our own sacrifice and gift.

What sustains us gives us the energy (Shakti) to take form and act. Understanding this, we understand that all that begins or is created must be sustained, or it ceases to be. This includes distress: understanding distress is sustained, and how, is essential to ending that distress.

Parvati

The Srimad Deva Bhagavatam describes the birth of Parvati. It is interesting to note that Parvati was born "after" many events had occurred which She caused. However, this illuminates a causality that does not apply to beings which exist beyond space and time, beyond form: to Shakti there is not "before" or "after."

The name of Parvati connotes a rock, or stone - as the daughter of the mountains or even the Shiva Lingam; it connotes what is beyond (para-), what fulfills and fills and is suitable (parv-), what was asked for or begged (-vati).

Sati's body had just been burnt; her true nature as Shakti was not known. Sati was Shiva's first wife, and to Shiva appeared to be mortal. The word "Sati" means "awareness" or "skillful attentiveness." Shiva was grieving. Shiva carried the partially cremated body about, utterly senseless. He meditated upon upon the form of Sati. Shiva's Samadhi was so profound that it first held everything still, and then reversed the paths, even of of the planets - the oceans stilled and began to merge with the mountains and islands and sky. The world was without joy, all beings were anxious or indifferent. This led to sorrow, and disease. The gods - and all beings - had their natures reversed, as if they had passed through a mirror of the soul.

At this time, a great Asura, named Taraka, received a gift from Brahma and became invincible. He conquered every world, and became rule of the universe. But the terms of the gift were not without exception (gifts from Brahma typically included at least one exception, since Brahma cannot give any extremity, not being an extremity himself): Taraka would remain invincible, except against the son of Shiva. Taraka knew that Shiva's wife had died, and he had no son - and would marry no other being. Taraka, remembering the ancient animosity between the Devas and the Asuras, punished the Devas severely. The Devas wept, and could see no end to their distress: "Shiva has no wife! How can he then have a son?"

Vishnu observed the distress of the Devas and learned of what Taraka had done. Vishnu assured the Devas, "do not be anxious, Shakti is aware of your distress. It is merely due to your faults that She shows Her indifference - Her indifference is meant to teach you, not destroy you. When a mother frightens and reprimands a child, it is not that she has became merciless; so will Shakti never be merciless to you. A child commits an offense if they do not live up to their mother's expectations; so too must you take refuge in Shakti, by improving yourselves." Vishnu, with his consort, Laxmi, then demonstrated to the Devas how to undertake the improvement required of them by Shakti. "You lack devotion," instructed Vishnu. High in the mountains, Vishnu taught the Devas Bhakti Yoga. Vishnu then taught them how to use mantra, combined with sacrificial action.

Soon, the Devas were improved sufficiently to recognize their numerous faults, and taking vows of self-improvement, held those vows. In this way, they emulated Shakti, and achieved Her expectations. The mantras were soon repeated constantly, their minds became singly focused, their action singly focused, and supreme sacrifices were made: the worst parts of their nature were painfully given up.

Soon, the Devas began to understand the true nature of Shakti; they no longer required sleep or rest. Over many years they became enlightened beings, and their enlightenment illuminated Shakti - right before them, among them. Together, they birthed Shakti. Shakti was as bright as lightning, red, cool like the moon, lustrous like the sun: the melody of the Vedas were personified in Her. There was fire above, below, on all sides - even in the middle. The fire had no beginning or end, but ignited the entire world.

In the midst of that light, the Devas were able to see Shakti: not as a woman, not as a man, not as a Deva, nor an Asura, nor any kind of Being. Then Shakti took form: Shakti became it became female, and a Deva - an exceedingly beautiful Deva. She was wearing beautiful and rich jewels, which shown in Her light. She wore ornaments on her waist and ankles, which tinkled as she walked. The smell of perfume enlivened the senses. On her forehead there was the sign of the half-crescent of Shiva. Her hair sparkled in the firelight. Her eyes sparkled in the firelight. The Puranas use many words to describe her beauty: she was the embodiment of awareness - holy allurement. She was Samadhi itself.

The Devas choked on tears of joy, they praised Her, and sang sweetly to Her, praising Her, loving Her devotedly. For they had by self-improvement become capable of that devoted love. And She loved them in return, with devoted love. Shakti was no longer Sati, but Parvati.

The Himalaya Mountains saw Parvati among the Devas, and asked Parvati to teach Bhakti Yoga. Parvati said,

Bhakti Yoga is the easiest path to Moksha, for it requires no hardship to the body, and merely bringing the mind to perfection through devoted, loving, venerating concentration. There are three practices of Bhakti.

Tamasic. A Tamasi will venerate Me with the intention of harming others, motivated by vanity, jealousy and anger: the Tamasi believes not only that I am different than They, but They are one among many individuals: they would not harm themselves, or Me.

Rajastic. Rajastic Bhakti is the veneration of Me for selfish welfare, without intending harm to others - but intending some desire or gain or enjoyment as the fruit of the practice: such a person perceives Me with duality, thinking disparity exists between Me and them when none actually exists.

Sattvic. Sattviki Bhakti is undertaken with the purpose of purification, when a person offers Me their own impurities by self-improvement. Giving me the result of all their Karmas, again they think that I am different than they. But the Sattviki makes the additional mistake of believing that just because such an offering is authorized in the Vedas it must be accepted. It need not be.

However, only a Sattviki can attain pure love, Parabhakti, supreme Bhakti.

The reason why Sattviki is the only path to Moksha is that only a person who does not possess the least desire to obtain the fruits of Bhakti, who does not desire liberation, will be sufficiently free of desire to obtain liberation: it is easy to become attached to the self-improving. However, the desire for liberation is the vehicle by which all other desires are let go. The means of letting go this last desire is to separate the duty of service from the servant; love must utterly consume their duty. Seeing Me everywhere, manifested in all, the devotee even sees Me in themselves. Everything fuels the passion of such true love. They become a lover - of all. In such a state of pure love, they become utterly selfless, and every act becomes one of devoted Bhakti. Every duty becomes a ritualized act of worship of Me. Karma Yoga and Bhakti Yoga become the same. Only then does such a worshiper forget concern for their preservation from past karmas, the desire for purification - because they have become purified.

In this state of purity, all action is Bhakti Yoga, and all Bhakti Yoga becomes an act of Jnana Yoga: knowledge of Me is obtained by every act, by every interaction, limitless knowledge results. Having become enlightened, the devotee is able to attain their final liberation.

Know, oh Mountain, that it is very difficult for any non-human being to perfect Bhakti Yoga, due to their nature. But it is very easy for any human being to attain the perfection of Bhakti. If a human being does not attain perfect Bhakti, it is because of some great calamity: for it is human nature to self-improve, to sacrifice, to let go of even letting go.

Book 7 Chapter 40 Srimad Devi Bhagavatam: Manifesting Parvati

Parvati said that She is manifested by waking and getting out of bed early (earlier than one normally wakes). At this point, like a thousand lotuses, the foremost of your mind should be filled with memory of your beloved, at their moment when they were most beautiful, with their consort(s) and/or attendant(s) (including you); fill yourself with love and admiration. This will permit you to take refuge in the highest Shakti Kundalini (latent energy), the Dharma of consciousness, manifested as Chaityana (consciousness of objectification) up-going the Brahmarandra (sensation of sensation, the apertures of the self), filled with awareness of the beloved: in other words, remembering your beloved at their most beautiful permits you to objectify them, idolize them, and use the energy of your idolization. This energy is the manifestation of the blissful nature of Parvati; the desire to merge with the beloved raises awareness of the separation required to serve the beloved.

Now, become aware of your separateness. Take care of your self, as you are important to your beloved: answer the calls of nature, bathe, complete Sandhya, Bandanams and other duties. This is the Agnihortra Homa (ritualized sacrificial gift of nutrient, commonly undertaken twice per day) to Parvati. This is the way Sankalapa (more than the vow or determination required to perform Puja, it is the architecture of the conditions required for success) is matured. Next, purify the the elements of your body (perform Bhuta Suddhi: mastering karma, so that your past need not fully dictate your future; it is here performed as a pause, a break) by respiration, arrange the letters and sounds of the mantra to master Maya (become free and in control of its illusion) to execute the Hrillekha Matrika Nyasa: I am every form of Matrika, every female form, every consort, the act of consorting. Devote every part of your body, every element of your form, every one of your forms to me in Nyasa. Finishing the Nyasas, it becomes understood that you are surrounded by paths of adharma, ajnana, avairagyam, ariddhi - each are like the compass directions themselves, leading toward you, leading you toward Dharma, Jnana, Vairagyam and Riddhi. Like a mountain, the world lies under your feet; like a mountain, you are master of Brahma, Vishnu, Shiva, Sadasiva and Isvara. You are where you should be at this moment, the end of your paths.

The elements of existence will become blurred into waking, dreaming, deep sleep, the higher jnanas; the jnanas are achieved, and you become aware of Brahma as I am, the consort of every existence, the force of form. This will inspire Japa: recite My name slowly, make a reminder of Me for yourself when your strength falters and you fail your Japa. This idol should be sprinkled with the sound of exasperation and exhaustion ("Phat" or "Phut") as the Japa fails; close the ten worlds by venerating your beloved. Meditate on your veneration until you find that it is love, then offer the gifts and sacrifices, your service of devotion. Meditate on attendance by contemplating the nature of Prabha (illumination) which occurs through devoted service. Then you will be ready to serve all beings as your beloved, as I serve all beings.

Enthralled with joy, every act of service and duty is cause for dance and singing: this glorifies the Veda Parayana, for it sacrifices your everything with your body to joy.

You will feed the Brahmanas, the Brahmacharis, the rich and the poor, thinking them all so many forms of your beloved; having manifested Me, you will see yourself as Me, your beloved as Me. Every being will bow before you, as they would to Me, for they will see you as Me. Merging with Me from your separateness, by your service, you will realize all which is possible, and eventually attain every goal you strive for.

Hrim is the essence of My mantra; like the many animals which live in the Ganges become part of its holiness and cause its holiness, and are the Ganges itself. If you can only do this once per week, Friday is the best day for it. Consider the meaning and purpose of these rituals, and you will understand how to adapt the practice to your particular Adhikara (claim), attaining your goal.

It is impossible to teach this ritual to those who are my enemies, or those who are cunning. As only a baby will nurse from their mother's breast (whether adopted or by birth), it is as useless and wrong to reveal this ritual to those who bear enmity to any other being as it would be to uncover a mother's breast to any but her baby, for neither baby nor mother will consent to the nursing. My disciples, My Bhaktas, are like the favorite child to me. I am like the mother of a household, rising early to serve Her family. Such service manifests good will, beauty, and devotion.

What is the goal, the purpose of this ritual? My manifestation (Parvati) will become Gauri, and Shiva loves Her, as She had been, as She was, as She would become, in all forms, always changing, never changing. Kartikeya (Parvati's son) was born of this constant love, and took form as a Deva, like His mother. Kartikeya destroyed the Tadaka Asura, because of such love, even before Gauri was known.

Parvati-Kali-Gauri

Parvati loved Shiva dearly. She was the manifestation of Sati's devotion. Though Shiva and Parvati had a son and lived eternities happily together, trouble began after Parvati defended Shiva from His enemies in battle: he had been overcome, and out of love she rushed to Shiva's defense.

But in her war, by degrees, she became enraged, and quite insane. She began to wear the heads of Her slain enemies about her neck, a skirt made of severed arms, and covered herself in gore; lighting fire to everything, she herself was scorched. she had to become fearsome, that her enemies would willingly submit to her, and stop harming Shiva. She began to delight in destruction!

But even after all her enemies were conquered, she was still so angry. She still delighted in destruction, and gore. She grew paranoid and violent; she saw enemies everywhere! She began to destroy everything! And even hurt herself! Everyone was terrified of her.

Because Shiva was the strongest, and her husband, and she might still love him, and not hurt him, even listen to him, Shiva was asked by every living being to restrain her. Yet Shiva knew she was stronger than him; Parvati was Shakti. Only she could restrain herself. But she was destroying everything she cared for, the entire world. So he had to do what could be done.

He approached her, and found she was ready to kill him, as well - Shiva, her true love, the one she had just saved! They were two halves of the same being, but in her insanity, she attacked Shiva. It was a difficult fight: She was well armed, and a trained fighter. At first, he blocked all her blows. Then, coming close to her, he held her in his arms, embracing her with love; in that embrace, Shiva tried to remind her who he was, who she was, to remind her of love. He bent time and space to imprison her, and tried to hold her still for a moment... and for a moment, she would seem to collect Herself - yet the instant he loosened his grip, she would again attack him. Again he would embrace her, and imprison her - and again, for a moment, she would regain self-control, only to lose it again.

In their battle, she struck him and hurt him in so many ways. They strove for what seemed an eternity; it was misery itself. She did not want to hurt him, and he did not want to hurt her; neither wanted to strive against the other - but she was not in control of herself. She was in a rage. After some time Shiva had to accept the fact that war left Parvati utterly insane.

Even today, you may know soldiers who do not come back from war the same way they left, or even wholly in their minds; or those whose troubled pasts or childhoods leave them insane and violent. Post-traumatic stress can destroy a person. She had been similarly injured by her war. She felt no grief at the hurt she caused Shiva, or the world. Shiva was not insane, and so did feel grief. This grief weakened Shiva more and more. Eventually, she was so much stronger than Shiva! Shiva began to weep, and was no longer able to fight.

Her fury grew as Shiva's weakness became evident: She was relying on Shiva to restrain Her; She had thought Him so strong! She admired His strength, and needed to believe He was invincible! Shiva persisted; but knew that He would be destroyed by Her before much longer. Everyone urged Shiva to kill Her in self-defense - but Shiva knew to do so would be to kill Himself. He was urged to kill Her in self-defense, in defense of the world, even if it destroyed Himself. They shared but one heart. This was the only hope for the world.

Shiva understood what He had to do - but could not bring himself to hurt his love, Parvati. He could not commit suicide, either (which would have destroyed Parvati, since they shared one heart). So, to save the world from her destruction, Shiva laid down before her, and permitted her to kill him - and thus bring about her own destruction.

Shiva laid himself down before her altar in supreme sacrifice. She gladly accepted the gift. She raised her sword for the victory blow, and then saw Shiva was weeping like a baby - for her impending death, grieving for their love. And at that moment, she shared his grief. She threw down all her weapons and wept with Shiva.

Shiva and Parvati held each other for a long time. She was scorched from battle, even Her hair was singed. Shiva held her in both hands and smiled, then laughed. She asked what Shiva was laughing at? Shiva pointed at her blackened skin, and in the emotional moment could only say "Kali!" The word encompassed the "black" color of her skin, the "grief" they both shared, the "one" heart they shared, the "strife" and "war" they had just shared, but it also carried the derogatory connotation of "imperfection," and "ugly."

She looked at herself and saw the filth that covered Her - not only the gore from Her war, but Shiva's own blood and tears. She saw where she had hurt Herself. She did not laugh. She was horrified, and desired to purify herself. She was no longer Parvati! She was Kali! Couldn't Shiva make her Parvati again? If Shiva could have given her that grace, he would have: but no one can escape the consequences of their actions, good or bad. Shiva forgave her, and urged her to forgive herself: She had been out of her mind and not responsible for her actions. Everyone - every being, even non-beings like she and Shiva - makes mistakes. But what she had done was necessary, a duty, and no mistake. The important thing was to recover, and do better. What was past could not be undone, but the future lay ahead. he loved her as Sati, he loved her as Parvati, he loved her as Kali.

This did not comfort her; She was overcome by regret, and felt too weak to do better. So She wept. From these tears were borne the Thugs, and all Criminal Yogis, whose Dharma is "black." Whose duty is "black."

Shiva tried to comfort her. She would not be comforted: She felt like she still had enemies to slay. Already, She felt the insanity growing again. Shiva urged her to forgive her enemies. But she was becoming gripped by insanity again, and could not. She warned Shiva, She would attack him again. She asked him to feel no remorse if he hurt her. So she and Shiva began to struggle again, but now Shiva felt no grief. Shiva defended Himself with all his strength, understanding compassion would require him to harm Kali. His great strength prevented her aggression from hurting Him - or the world. And woke her to her own weakness. Suddenly, she regained self-control again.

When the fit had passed, She understood how the war had wounded Her. She understood at that moment She could no longer be Shiva's Wife, or his friend, nor be near anything she loved; She could perform no duty. She had no reason to live; She would hurt anything near her or dear to her. She vowed she would destroy Herself upon Shiva's altar, for She had become his enemy, her own enemy. Death was better than that incurable injury which caused so much distress to her and those who cared for her.

Remembering when she had burned herself upon his altar in the form of Sati, Shiva held her close and wept. And as we wept a river of tears, all her Black was washed away - Kali was washed away! The Black took a hollow form and, possessed of insanity and wrath, tried to hurt Shiva, but was powerless. The hollow Kali then tried to destroy the world, but was powerless. The hollow Kali then fled across every world, in impotent anger and fury. This hollow Kali was Kausiki: hollowness and without form, pure power, without mind, heart or body, a pure selfish malice, devoid of love. No longer His wife, Kausiki left Shiva's presence. He was glad when Kausiki left.

When Kausiki left, what was left of Kali was Gauri: the body, heart and mind underneath that shell of blackness. All that Black shell had been washed away by tears, and utterly purified! This was pure reflected Shakti, and she was radiant! Kali was no more.

Gauri stood before Shiva; her skin as white as if she had never seen the sun in all her life. Indeed, She had been there all along, under that Black skin. Behind all that blackness. His wife had forgotten who She truly was: not Kali, not Parvati, not even Sati. But Shiva remembered when he wept. And this grief manifested his understanding of Shakti; Shakti had taken form before Shiva, as Gauri, by this devotion. Now, Shakti was embodied in a more perfected form, as Gauri. Gauri was everything Shakti wanted to become. She embraced Shiva, and at that moment taught Shiva to let go of all the pain He still held in His heart for Sati, Parvati and Kali; when his profound distress from sympathy in Kali's suffering was extinguished, he learned better wisdom.

Ardhanarishwara

Gauri is a manifestation of Shiva's love for Shakti: Gauri is the reflection of every form of Shakti. Therefore, as Shiva is the only one to truly know Shakti, Gauri is as close a conception as can be made of Shakti using form: an indirect inference must sometimes suffice for an inability for direct observation; a mirror image may permit the sight of what is behind, and out of direct sight.

The mother of Ganesh is celebrated through Swarna Gauri Vratha, a day before Ganesh Chaturthi (remembering how Gauri created Ganesh - Ganesh is the reflection of Gauri's love for Shiva). It is a day traditionally set aside for devotions to be made to one's spouse, or for the desiring of a spouse to be known. It is typical to visit in-laws and be served special foods, so they can celebrate the marriage. It used to be customary for a newly-wed couple to wait until Swarna Gauri Vratha to first attempt pregnancy: this was done because a child would be born 9 months later in summer, when it would be more likely to survive due to environmental concerns.

Gauri attempted to make herself worthy of Shiva's love, through devotional Yoga. For 16 years, She practiced perfectly. Shiva noticed Gauri, and asked Gauri what it was that she desired from his love. She said that she desired nothing less than to be Shiva's Ardhangini, and that Shiva would have no other wife but her. She wanted Shiva to love her as she loved him, constantly, purely, and solely. She made profound vows. Shiva was touched, and agreed, "I shall have not even the thought of another in my heart but you." Shiva laid his heart bare for Gauri to see, and it was like a mirror: she saw only her own image in it. Gauri was so happy, she knelt down before Shiva, and crying with joy, gave thanks. Shiva lifted her up, and held her tightly: She was his Ardhangini, half of his being - and should not bow before him. They rejoiced together for a very long time. "Eternities came and went."

One day, Shiva sat on a rock in Kailasa, and Gauri was sitting beside Him; She was so happy because she was with Him. And then, all of a sudden, everything seemed wrong to Gauri. She actually began to tremble with fear, doubt, anguish. All her strength left Her, She grew limp and felt weakness like a poison pushed through Her veins by Her heart. She saw in Shiva's heart not Her own reflection, but the image of another! A beautiful Deva! Oh, Gauri was so jealous! This Deva was beautiful, more beautiful than She ever could be! Young, desirable - and in the same joyous love Gauri had known. This woman was beloved of Shiva! Jealousy became hatred. And because both Shiva and Gauri shared one heart, the poison passed through Shiva's body, and He began to suffer as well.

Beyond time, beyond space, the two sank into misery. Gauri began to doubt that She kept her vows, for why else would Shiva have broken His? She knew though that she had kept every promise. She faded from existence, and Shiva lost his own breath; the two were one, inseparably one. Like fish need water, Shiva could not survive. Shiva sought in every world. Eventually, on a mountaintop, in a world of darkness, the ghost of Gauri sat - no happiness existed in her; She was consumed by desire, aversion, hatred.

Shiva took her in His arms, so glad to have found her. He pressed her close to his heart, and she began to breathe again. He asked her, "what had happened? Why had she become so tormented?" He kissed her forehead, her cheeks, her lips, her head; he called out her name over and over again. Gauri! Gauri! But she could not respond, she was consumed by despair. And so Shiva wept. And as his heart began to break, Gauri's own heart felt pain. The pain woke her a little, her spirit form was in agony. She held Shiva closer, and felt life; She began to feel terror - at losing Shiva. Then She remembered that other woman in Shiva's heart - and violently pushed Shiva away from Her and in an angry tirade explained how Shiva had been so cruel to Her, how he had made her existence meaningless and destroyed Her. And she ripped open his chest to lay bare his heart.

But it was her face she saw in the heart. Both she and Shiva now wept. She asked what happened to the other woman who was in his heart, but now was not there? The woman who had taken her place in Shiva's heart?

Shiva stopped weeping a moment. Then, understanding what had happened, smiled. Then he laughed. "Her?" He laughed louder and louder, increasingly relieved - "Her?" it seemed so cruel to Gauri. The beautiful woman's face was again in Shiva's heart. "Look - it is Parvati. It is your own reflection!" Shiva laughed.

Gauri felt confused, then understood. Then she was embarrassed a moment. But then She too, smiled. And laughed at her own foolishness. In an instant She and Shiva were sitting in Kailasa again, the sun was shining just as before - there was no regret: beyond time, beyond space, it did not matter how long the two had been in misery - they were now happy again. As if they had always been happy. And she saw her beautiful smile in the reflection. In Shiva's heart. And laughed with relief and happiness.

Shiva then made a promise to Gauri, that this would never happen again. "From now on, you and I shall not be Ardhanginis, two bodies with a single heart, but a single united body." They embraced, and in that hug held each other so tightly that the two became one. By devotional Bhakti, they became a half-male, half-female Ardhanarishwara.

Durga

There is enormous variation in the practice of Durga Puja, but the study, veneration by emulation, and reverence of Durga is central to all.

Just as Brahma, Shiva and Vishnu represent three manifestations of form, and there are many other forms besides these, Shakti is manifested by numerous forces, powers and energies - but principally as the consort of Brahma, half of Shiva, the Ardhangani of Vishnu, the wives of Ganesh, etc. etc. Durga represents not only the combination of all forces, powers and energies, but the manifestation of their form: she is the combination of Brahma, Shiva and Vishnu - as well as Saraswati, Gauri, and Laxmi. As well as all other beings and non-beings. She is the union of all, good and evil.

Durga is a word that implies a fortress, a defensible position which is invincible. She describes herself as the bending of Shiva's bow, implying the act itself as well as its intention, and all precedent training, and the asana. She describes herself as both father and mother, implying the creative act of not only copulation, but rearing. She describes Herself as consciousness itself. She is known as the Buffalo Slayer, the death of Death, the corruptor of Corruption, the end of Endings. She is known as the All-Woman, the embodiment of femininity. Even the femininity present in masculinity (the two are not wholly distinct).

The reason all beings and non-beings manifested this union Durga was the necessity to defend themselves against destruction and obstruction. It is difficult to imagine a force countering all Dharma, Adharma and Non-Dharma alike, yet this was Durga's enemy. Words are important to conception, so the words "perversely unnatural" (what corrupts a thing's nature) and "betrayal" and "sabotage" (counter-duty, counter-loyalty) may be used, as may "de-loving" (not so much hate, nor unloving, but corruptive of love). "Self-destructive" is also a good term, especially when it is understood that something truly self-destructive will destroy all of its environment with it as well. Derelict in duty.

Durga's enemy began existence as an Asura, who decided to perpetuate the war between the Devas and the Asuras. Rambha, the King of the Asuras, had fallen in love with a water buffalo and married her. Their daughter was called Mahishi, and their son was called Mahishasura, which means "water buffalo asura."

Mahishasura, before beginning his campaign against the Devas, asked Brahma for a gift of invincibility. But Brahma, instead offered that Mahishasura would only be in danger from being harmed by women. This was good enough for Mahishasura, as he did not believe any woman could withstand his strength. Or his sex appeal. Mahishasura then began a terrible campaign, which threatened to destroy Dharma itself. He knew no restraint, and even hurt himself, knowing that he could not destroy himself (he could only be endangered by a woman). Things got pretty horrific.

Durga, being the ultimate feminine, (and by nature, the union of all beings, also all women), ultimately killed Mahishasura after a long battle, in which he came to regret his gift from Brahma, regret his war against the Devas, and love Durga, regretting his battle against her. More, in the battle, Durga destroyed the self-destructive tendencies of both the Asuras and Devas, bringing an end to their war.

The story relates numerous shape-shifting by both Durga and Mahishasura, all of which recalls progressions of Asanas. Durga is the bow of shiva, and also the Asana of the bow; Durga is the tree which withstands the buffalo's wrath, and also the Asana of the tree. And so forth. Being all forms, all energies, a Yogi may learn to freely transition between Dharmas, natures and duties, to accomplish their purpose. This is true Hatha Yoga. To a Yogi, there is no masculine or feminine, nor any caste; all is embodied as one. As Durga.

Sita

Sita, perceiving Parvati, understanding their shared being, bowed low and said,

Oh, Parvati, you saw Shiva, and loved Him, but he did not see you, nor could he love you if he did - not wholly as the partridge sees and loves the moon, for you shine too, and are worthy of that love you desired. Ganesh and Kartikeya are not your only children: you have been the mother to every being. Beyond time, beyond eternity, beyond the Vedas, beyond depth, the co-condition of existence and non-existence, your play is with all creation. You entice, you are the motivation. Merely seeing you has led to the greatest satisfaction, all beings bow down before you, and are content. You know my heart's desire, it is your heart, and your desire too. Within that heart we share, within that desire we share, we never part: I need not speak my thoughts, for they are yours.

Parvati, perceiving Sita, understanding their shared being, smiled and placed a flower necklace around Sita's neck to honor Her. When Sita accepted the honor, Parvati was filled with joy, and happiness, and said,

Oh, Sita, I will speak my thoughts, because they are yours. Be assured. What you desire is also already yours; the discomfort you feel is merely your desire, not the wanting of it.

Narada always speaks words pure and true: He whom you desire will be your husband.

Maya

When Shakti first manifested as Parvati, she said to all the beings gathered about her,

Realize who and what I am. I am beyond existence, beyond mind, beyond thought, beyond name, beyond birth, beyond death, beyond form. Like Maya, I am not existent, nor non-existent, neither existent nor non-existent, nor both existent nor non-existent. I am known as Chit, Shambit, Para Brahma, and many other names. Is the light which comes from the sun the sun itself? Is the light of the moon the moon itself? Who and what I am cannot be seen because of the form it manifests. Know that I am the cause of being, I am like Maya, the cause of all form. Like Maya is ended by Jnana Yoga without destruction, I, too have ended, and am beyond ending.

Editorial note: Maya is a word which comes from the root "man-" meaning "to think:" the Buddha Gotama taught that an observer and reality are co-originating – that an observer affects what they are observing by their observation. What is seen, heard, touched, tasted and felt are subject to interpretation; the world is only as we think we have observed it. When Brahma discovered this principle, numerous forms of Brahma were manifested, to interact with what was being observed, to preserve and protect what was being observed from being affected by that observation, etc. The Buddha was nearly conquered by Mara (a masculine form of Maya), but after struggle, conquered Mara; Maya also was the mother of the Buddha - in this way, Maya is symbolically presented as the theory and practice of Buddhist Jnana yoga. It is because we are subjected to such bias that we overcome it.

Parvati continued: Maya is twofold: Avidya (the belief in disparity between form and reality, observer and observed) and Vidya (the belief that observer and observed are the same, the unity of form and reality): Avidya permits truth to be hidden, and Vidya permits truth to be found. The force which brings interaction between observer and observed is both distinct from both observer and observed, and because it is organized wholly dependent upon both observer and observed - while simultaneously self-organized, it is incorrect to describe it as distinct or indistinct. When two beings love each other so truly that the love shapes their nature, can the love be said to be distinct from their nature? Is a child the product of only one parent, or the other - or neither, or both? Is an infant in the womb distinct or indistinct from their mother? In this way, I am the cause and the effect of all being.

Intelligence is self-organizing, there can be no specific cause for that intelligence which is discovered: in the same way, the sun is self-illuminating (though beyond the anticipation of the ancient text, a modern analogy is provided in the same context: the sun's light self-organizes after sufficient mass is accumulated to result in sustained nuclear fusion - though fusion was beyond the ancient understanding, a similar concept based upon an atomic theory of matter formed the same basic premise). It is this process of self-organization which I am. The sun's light illuminates other objects, but these, though touched by the sun, are not the sun. Intelligence is everlasting: Waking or dreaming, living in one form or another, we retain our identity, though connected - such retaining is what I am.

Jnana Yoga is the means by which intelligence is explored, sensed and understood. Intelligence is understood to be the nature of Love. I am Love. Love is the only sensation intelligence is capable of discerning: as darkness is only the absence of light, intelligence is only able to discern the absence of Love - or its presence. Love is continuous: there are a multitude of degrees and purities of love. So is intelligence: intelligence exists simultaneously in every degree and purity. Jnana is not the Dharma, but it is the nature of Atman: Atman is not the Dharma. Jnana is the result of intelligence aware of intelligence, it is self-awareness. Yet the observation of the self affects the self. Intelligence is not the Dharma. Form is not different from the form used to observe that form. Atman only exists when united with Maya.

Awakening is therefore impossible through intelligence. What is real is not manifested like form, nor can intelligence realize or manifest Atman. Only what is unaffected by observation, unmanifested by intelligence, is real. Reality can only be logically inferred - as what is without form is inferred by what has form. A hole is only known through the material surrounding it. I am this act of inference.

When will, intelligence and action become one, sight, sound, touch, taste, smell and all perception result in the strings (Sutras) of sensuality: these strings bind existence, and give it a nature, a "Sutratman" called

"Linga Deha." This is composed of all the Pranas, resulting in the Causal Body. Yet the organs which see, smell, hear, taste and touch are composed of the same materials they are observing, and the materials are continuous and contiguous. This continuity, this contiguity is a type of Cosmic Body (Virat). The nature of the connection between all matter self-organizes as a result of matter. It is this process of self-organization which I am.

When a refugee takes refuge in themselves, I am that refugee's strength. With sufficient strength of mind, body and heart, reality may be observed by reflection, as if distantly through a mirror: those strong of mind, body and heart are the mirror. Only the strength itself is real. The mirror may reflect an image, but it does not contain what it is reflecting. No more than a rope mistaken as a snake could present any real danger. The strength of this form, the potency of the illusion I present by this form, is not Me; but it does distantly reflect Me.

Artha Veda VII 50 - The Victory

That ancient tree weathered countless storms only to be utterly destroyed by the chance strike of a single bolt of lighting. Thus may I hope to win with the roll of my dice against my opponents. Whether my opponents are prepared, ready and alert (or not) matters nothing to my luck: that ancient tree was strong, too, and had survived so many storms and attacks. My opponent will not defend themselves against me any better for their many advantages than that ancient tree could resist Indra's lighting bolt.

See how my enemies already are assembled on all sides? They now move against me - they think this is their chance, for I am caught, at disadvantage, outmatched and outnumbered! They think this their chance - but "chance" is not theirs to possess. Indeed, it may be MY chance. Perhaps now I shall take back what is mine! Indeed, they owe me a great debt, having injured me so. Look how they gather about me - bringing back what was mine to retake in victory!

It is true, I am weaponless. My hands are empty, they have disarmed me. Yet though I may be weaponless I am not defenseless. An empty hand never remains empty long. The hand which is empty may more easily grasp and take hold than the one which holds too much - and they hold what is mine, besides their own. Overburdened, they shall not easily defend themselves, or what they wrongly hold.

At this moment I reflect that I have always fed Agni's sacrificial fire. Indeed, I have given all I have to Agni. Has my sacrifice been enough to satisfy Agni? Agni's sacrificial fire can be fed, constantly, and without satisfaction. Always desiring, always hungry, Agni would consume all the wealth of the world - yet would hunger still for more. And if permitted to escape, He would not hesitate to consume anything in His path - for all is rightfully His. Can anything given to Agni be taken back? Nothing given to Agni can ever be taken back, for He burns it utterly to ash. Agni hungers for everything, acquires everything and defends forever. As I shall. Through patience and generosity toward my opponents, I have sacrificed all I have to Agni. And now I have become as hungry as Fire itself!

I have by such devotion of patience and generosity toward my opponent given all to Agni. Thus have I manifested that sacred Fire within Me. Look, I am now like Agni Himself! If permitted the opportunity, I shall, too, acquire and defend. I shall, too, succeed - as Agni always accomplishes the sacrifice required by destroying what is given upon the altar. So now shall I accomplish the sacrifice required of my opponents! They shall feed my fire, they shall atone! They shall give to Agni! They shall feed my fire, and seek the Marutaganas, those Rudras who by the command of Indra make the rain fall to extinguish the fires of Agni. But the Marutaganas can come only after Agni has taken what is His. I shall take what is mine before being made to desist. I shall give a reason for it to rain!

Indra's lightning, striking an ancient tree, can spark Agni's fire. Oh, how I was struck by my enemy! Yet from the fire of a single bolt of Indra's lightning, Agni can devour the entire forest, and ignite the world. Today this old tree burns. I burn, I am angry. Indra has lit my Fire, and prepared the sacrifice of my opponents. Indra has thus conquered my opponent's troops with fire. My opponents shall satisfy Agni, now they have lit the fire! I shall burn them all to ash. Oh, Maghavan! Oh, Indra! You make a path for me through these obstacles, and I am now like a charioteer running a race upon that road. Oh, Maghavan! You never remain defeated for long! So too will I rise from defeat to crush my enemies and conquer their troops!

As a wolf jealously defends Agni's fuel from the sheep who dare attack the holy plants so will I take what my enemies have wrongly won. I shall be a wolf among such hungry, insolent sheep! I will be as merciless as a gambler who cleans out his opponent, taking even the reserve funds. Does the lightning leave anything of the tree it strikes? A strong hand in cards does a player no good against a bold bluffer, and patience earns nothing for the one who waits too long to play his cards, thinking to heap up his winnings. The Gambler plays the game as his duty, his Dharma. The Gambler loves the game, despite the risk. The Gambler will not spare any money, nor fear losing it, for he can believe that playing the game with such duty will give him winnings as its justice. For the Gambler has faith that if he only perseveres a little longer, there will be justice, and he will win back what was his. The Gambler believes winning is his right, and is justice - am I wrong to trust in Justice as I now, too, roll the dice?

It is by wealth we suppress our wretched poverty, it is by grain we suppress our hunger (if only for a little while). So must we sometimes resort to perseverance and the cunning of audacity to suppress our misfortune. Gambling is now my work, my duty, my love and joy. It is my Artha, Dharma, and Kama. For I am desperate. Alas, that I am so desperate. Look, I now must wager greatly, or else lose everything anyway. Perhaps I now gamble foolishly? Though indeed it is likely I shall come to harm and misfortune, I am already harmed, and any further patience or non-action will result in my utter defeat. It is only by this gamble do I have the chance of victory.

Am I fool? The odds are against me. Only a fool seeks a strong opponent. Yet it is good reason that nothing is certain. Lightning strikes are not common, they are rare, they are unlikely - but do happen. Is it not also possible that the dice will provide and nourish me today? It was by chance that I was struck down. It is also possible I may strike a bit of luck too, and become bound up by it in a streak long enough for victory - even as the bows of my enemies are already bound up by string and directed against me!

So come now, give me the dice: the game is not yet over. Like a Sannyasi, like a Gambler, I lay all I have down - upon the table. I have one more play left and would indeed be a fool to leave the game just because of a little bad luck!

Week 5 and 6

SUMMARY

Beginner's Class: Introduction to the Dharma of Asanas. Introduction to Artha and Kama. Introduction to Sacrifice. Intermediate Class: Bhakti Yoga. Puja. Sacrifice of Animals. Vegetarianism. The relationship between theism, atheism and non-theism in yoga. Diwali. Vehicles. Kalki.

Training methods
- Understanding the concept of Dharma in terms of duty, or necessity,
    - Develop the understanding of the necessity for Asanas: the necessity of health, courtesy, friendship, companionship, family, business, work, all karma.
    - Develop from the dharma of karma, develop an understanding of Artha as a goal of practice.
    - Without enjoyment of what is earned, without sacrifice, without Kama, Artha cannot achieve Dharma.
- Theism, Atheism and Non-Theism are Ashramas, stages, in practice, preparing the yogi for the next stage. Freedom in movement between the three requires understanding their necessity and not attaching to belief or disbelief. What is achieved when these three are sacrificed: Dharma.

Introduction to Artha and Kama

Dharma is best observed and expressed in terms of duty, or necessity, and achieved in terms of expediency and efficiency. But these concepts require taking up, artificially adopting a goal. The most expedient and efficient path is measurable only when the beginning and end points are known, and the purpose of the journey is known too. The best path is not necessarily a straight line: one must arrive prepared to accomplish the purpose. Sometimes a person might stop along the way home from work to pick up food for dinner, or on the way to the temple to buy flowers as a sacrifice, or take a scenic route to arrive calm and centered. Or to ensure they do not arrive too early (which can be as deleterious as arriving too late).

The end of Dharma is Artha, and the purpose of Dharma is Kama.

Consider, do you not yet know the beginning - the reason why you practice Yoga? Or does this secret knowledge remain elusive? You are not alone: so many wander on, not remembering where they came from, forgetting even where they were headed, and for what purpose. You have wandered on in ignorance and sleep long enough: practice jnana, and awaken yourself.

For what purpose do you eat? Food suppresses hunger only a short while. For what purpose do you eat wholesome foods? Even the most healthy people have not lived much more than 130 years. Why exercise, why take care of yourself? Why do you develop friendship, family, career - only to give these up? Understanding karma, the yogi comes to understand (eventually) that any action which is not dharma has karma: result, effect, and cause: every action is co-conditioned by its effect. And desiring to be free of karma, seeks to practice only dharma. But this is not an escape.

The purpose of sacrifice is to prepare the yogi to sacrifice sacrificing. The Dharma itself must eventually be given up. When one can face karma fearlessly, then one may truly master it. This sacrifice of sacrifices is the end of Dharma: this courage is the essence of Artha, of work, and effort, of inducing karma.

Yet it is insufficient to merely not be afraid, to be brave and courageous. It is insufficient to work hard. What is produced must be enjoyed. Kama is purpose of Dharma, the end of Karma. Kama is the reason for which all beings venture forth into wandering. What is worked toward must achieve this reason. Kama is gained by yagna.

Mantra of Kama: "I can understand"

The Shiva Purana explains that after Kamadeva is born, in every re-creation, Kamadeva stands before Brahma and asks, "Kam darpayani?" "whom shall I please?" Brahma is not one to give a plain answer, but rather the means for you to discover the answer for yourself. So, Brahma says: "if you but arm yourself, even should your arrows be made of flowers, you will find no one – not even I – will able to be victorious against you. Yet you will not be undefeated." Om Kamadevaya. Vidmahe! Kamadeva followed the advice of Brahma, and quarreling with everyone, eventually came to say, Vidmahe, "I can understand." For having remained undefeated in every world, in every time, he then conquered himself. To do so, he pleased himself greatly.

Editor's notes:
- *The multiple meanings of many of the words and phrases permits extensive analysis of this passage. What is of special note to this text is that "I can understand" is also connotative of the understanding that comes with "regret" - especially in the sense of Artha...as in having worked for the wrong reasons, having worked in the wrong way, having failed to obtain satisfaction, having failed to succeed, having found no pleasure. Love, friendship, pleasure guides honorable effort.*
- *Kamadev is a fundamental avatara of Vishnu, and the Kalki purana, especially, presents the last (end, in the connotation of purpose) plays of Kamadev. This is why Kalki is accompanied by the parrot of this wisdom (Rati). The purpose (end) of of sacrifice is the sacrifice*

of sacrificing. The purpose (end, and beginning) of Vishnu, of the Dharma, is Kama.

What is Artha?

Artha cannot be translated simply, as it is a word founded in contextual reference that is utterly foreign to English, but is best understood through its relationship to Dharma and Kama. The end of Dharma is the means of Artha, the purpose of Dharma is Kama. It is the resource, skill of resourcefulness, the gain of resources, the use of resources. The necessary object of effort toward Kama, toward enjoyment. The means of life and living is not always the purpose of life and living, but the purpose of life and living permit many such means of life and living - this purpose is Kama.

Therefore, the closest approximation to Artha may be "acquisition," for it is the means by which Kama can be acquired from Dharma. And therefore, there is no single correct expression of Artha: for Dharma and Kama vary widely, depending on a person's karma.

In practicing asanas, Dharma is discovered first by practicing what is easy and hard, then understanding what is necessary. In practicing asanas, Artha is discovered by the process by which that which is necessary is achieved so that its benefit may be enjoyed: the way in which something is accomplished matters quite as much as the ultimate accomplishment of it. Even failure in the accomplishment can, if it is performed with honor, result in the enjoyment of that effort. If accomplished without honor, then even if the accomplishment succeeds, then it will not be enjoyed.

What is worked for must be enjoyed: Artha permits Dharma to achieve Kama. Kama is purpose of Dharma, the end of Karma. Kama is gained by yagna.

What is yagna / yajna? Puja?

Yajna is a particular form of sacrifice, one which will typically (but not always) utilize fire.

There are several forms of fire: the flame of combustion, the heat of gathering fuel for combustion, the knowledge (light) of the mind, the warmth of love or friendship, etc.

There are several forms of sacrifice: the using up, the destruction, the giving, the sharing, etc.

Every type of sacrifice is performed for honor: for the giver to gain honor, for the giver to give honor to the receiver, for the honor of both giver and receiver, to honor that which is sacrificed, etc. This honor, this puja, is accomplished by fire-sacrifice - in the same way that Dharma accomplishes Kama by Artha. The fire, and the sacrifice, together, are both important to the success of this particular puja.

Fire forces a particular action in sacrifice, namely devotion, confidence, fealty, loyalty: what is fed to the fire cannot be taken back. Understanding this secret knowledge permits use of other forms of fire than combustion, and greater sacrifices than combustibles. It is by such greater sacrifices on greater fires that Atman is discovered.

Yoga is the means by which these greater fires are kindled.

Do you not yet understand the means by which sacrifice is made on this yogic fire? Do you require priests (a kind of assistant to the one performing sacrifice) to assist you? There are several kinds of priests: those capable of assisting through encouragement, technical support, and agency. The Hotri priest is able to help because they have studied the Rigveda. The Adhvaryu is able to act in agency by ensuring the altar, fire and sacrifice are performed properly - having studied these. The Udgatri supports with encouragement, singing the Samaveda. The Brahmin can correct the mistakes which are likely to occur during complicated rituals like this, having understood what is actually important and essential (perfection is not the goal).

Agni (the fire) is the priest to Indra. Having kindled your own fire, can you not become your own priest? Having become a Brahmin, can you not correct your own mistakes? Can you not study the vedas, and the rituals? Do you not understand your purpose, and means?

Having manifested Agni and hearing Svaha calling you home, can you not manifest Indra, and hear Agni calling you to sacrifice?

Having manifested Indra, you can then perform the greatest Indra Pujas, including the manifestation of society, friendship, ardhangini, and children. This is why Yagna is the primary ritual of the bonds of friendship, or the bonding of families, of the social bondings of society, of the bonding of marriage.

The greatest Yagna of all, though, is the one for which no further Yagna is required. The greatest sacrifice is the sacrifice of sacrificing.

Yajnavalkya Upanishad: the greatest Yagna

The greatest Yagna is the one which accomplishes the purpose of Yagna, and brings an end to Yagna. The greatest sacrifice is the one which accomplishes the purpose of the sacrifices, necessitating no further sacrifice. The sacrifice of sacrifices is not the end of sacrifices, nor the purpose of sacrifice.

The purpose of learning geometry is not the knowledge of shape, but learning the construction of shape. In constructing shapes, knowledge emerges. It is in the same way that wisdom emerges from the temple: understanding shape permits understanding relationships, and this is the means to application. The sacred act of such geometry reveals what was perceived but not known: what is defined can be related, and such relation produces the conditions for what is desired. This is the way and reason for which an altar is constructed through geometry.

As one might become disgusted with life after their friend or spouse dies, discontinuing the fire ritual, or failing to maintain the fire, as a fire may be permitted to extinguish itself, so does that which sustains life bring an end to it.

Those who have sacrificed their semen to Indra [*either into fire, or into the uterus - editor*] find that the fire knows no difference between blood and water [connoting both the menstration signaling failed pregnancy (where is the semen in the blood?), and simultaneously the fire itself). The ashes of wood, grass, flesh, even fluids of many kinds are the same. What difference is there between the ashes of blood, saliva, mucus, bile, semen or any of the other liquids in the body when the water common in them all is removed? This is how by sacrifice one understands a great deal of impurity can be tolerated by Agni, how Agni takes all that is fed to it, all is the same to Agni in the end. Discover the limits of your own tolerance for impurity: it is not by wearing the sacred thread that one becomes a Brahaman, but by satisfying the conditions of confidence in your sacrifice. It is frequently good enough. Svaha!

How can one injure another when seeking for Brahma, in Brahmacharya? Even if one seeks Brahma upon the battle's field, you will not harm another, and in such harmlessness, succeed. Fast even unto your death, enter into the purifying waters until you drown: you will not destroy yourself. All limits or extremity are illusionary, yet there is nevertheless Brahma. Seek this Brahma not in the extremities, but in the exertion of the seeking. Then you will find Brahma in the sufficiency of your moderation and self-restraint, in the limits of reality. Indeed, one who collapses on their journey fails in it, but the one who takes it in stages (Ashramas) succeeds - and returns home.

Sages wear no distinguishing marks, and yet conduct themselves sensibly. Proclaim sufficiency! All you do teaches, speaks, tells of sufficiency! A child is born without clothes, as if unaffected by heat or cold, pleasure or pain, incapable of accepting anything. And yet this child will take up the wearing of clothing, even ceremonial clothing, only to discard it later. You are well-established in the path, incapable of avoiding the stages of your journey. By merely sustaining your life, you succeed.

Do you think Atman is in every being? Bow before all beings and you will soon give up that thought. Sacrifice that belief, and all others. Having bowed to every being, you will no longer bow before anyone. Nor tolerate any bowing before you. You neither require nor deserve to be bowed to.

There are those who sacrifice their fluids to Indra in the hope of a child. But this is not how children are gained. There are those who believe that a child will bring them happiness. But one quickly learns even a son who is unborn worries the parents: often, the mother and father worry for miscarriage and failure, even before the quickening. And once birth is successful, the son worries his parents that he will not learn, or thrive, or mature beyond the stage (Ashrama) of his parents and fail his purpose. And after his mother and father are dead, he then troubles himself: sometimes he might even fail because of the extent of his worrying. Bound and attached to the success he desires, even those desires of his parents, he becomes prisoner to the victory he desires. He avoids women, for fear of sexuality, and makes sacrifices to fires without ever achieving success - for he does not understand what it means to succeed. Having never embarked upon the journey, he does not know lies beyond the stages.

Theragatha 12.2: the better man

The monk Sunita said, I was born in a low caste, an outcaste. I was born poor, with next to no food. My work was degrading, I gathered whatever was spoiled. I gathered the withered flowers from the shrines and threw them away. People found me disgusting, despised me, disparaged me. I prostrated myself to show reverence to everyone, and even came to lower my heart.

But then one day, I saw the Buddha Gotama, arrayed with a squadron of monks, the great victorious hero, entering the city of the Magadhans. I threw down my carrying pole and hurried to show him my reverence. I prostrated myself to him. And he – the good man that he was – stood still out of sympathy – just for me!

Since he stood still for me, I rose, and stood before him. He then said, "come, monk!" And I then walked with my teacher.

Later, alone, I meditated in the wilds, untiring, following his instructions just as he taught me. And then I conquered, just as he, the Conqueror, had once conquered! Like him, it was in the first watch of the night that I remembered all my previous existences, in the middle watch, I was purified. And as the last watch ended, I burst through the mass of darkness like the sun!

And as I rose with the sun and went to visit my teacher, Indra and Brahma – whose wilted flowers I had once thrown away – came and knelt before me, praising me for my victory. And since I stood still for them, they stood before me, and then walked with me! Arrayed with a squadron of devas, I returned to my teacher, who, seeing me victorious, smiled when he saw me.

My teacher taught me it is not by birth that one is a high caste, a supreme man, a Brahman, praised by Indra and Brahma.

Through self-control and righteousness one becomes a better man.

Puja and Bhakti Yoga: Apara-Bhakti Yoga and Para-Bhakti Yoga

Beginning your practice of Bhakti begins by discovering those qualities which are honorable in yourself, so they may developed. This is accomplished by recognizeed those qualities in others for emulation. This is accomplished by understanding the form or effect of these qualities through Apara-Bhakti so their cause may be discerned.

Eventually, by Para-Bhakti, the Yogi sees these qualities everywhere - because they have manifested these qualities within themselves – and understands that it is their perception of these qualities which manifests them in others. When the Bhakti sees honor everywhere, their training has been successful and they are ready for practice, and performance.

During training, it is recommended that a person become sectarian, devoted to a single teacher. Most Yogis never progress beyond this stage because their teacher has not progressed beyond this stage. The teacher, upon observing sectarian and singularity of devotion, should recognize their student is ready to progress - and help them, by friendship through Sat-sang, to accomplish the sacrifice of the teacher.

Eventually, the student should surpass their teacher in some way or another and discover their own capacity to teach in some way or another, and then understand equality. A book has a back cover, but is not discarded upon completion: the student must become worthy of the sacrifices of their teacher, and give the gifts of friendship.

The yogi then seeks other teachers, and builds friendship between them.

Consider, a flower is an object first for venerating, then of veneration. A spouse is loved, a flower given to them: then the flower is itself loved as much as a spouse, as a reflection of their love. A flower is loved through cultivation, and in the wild, in admiration.

Any being, every being, can be a teacher. The Bhakti builds friendship between all beings. All beings can learn and practice Bhakti yoga.

In your training, discover faults and failings in your teacher. A student will first see these as dishonor, but it is a natural development of their own Bhakti: can you see the faults of another, and still honor and love them?

These faults force us to turn away from the teacher, and seek others. By seeking others we see the entire world is full of faults. Then, by further study, we learn that these faults are actually evidence of perfection: our conception of perfection is illusionary. We would not see fault if we did not imagine perfection. And then to see perfection.

Awaken a perfected love: unconditional, loyal, universal, total. It is by Bhakti, through the process of honoring, then finding fault, that fault is destroyed by love, Prem.

As with any other path of Yoga, every action must train and practice Bhakti. As the practice of Puja develops and advances, it expands to include every action. And every action inspires Bhava, the feeling of devoted love, worship, veneration.

Swami Sivananda teaches, "there are five kinds of Bhava in Bhakti. They are Shanta, Dasya, Sakhya, Vatsalya and Madhurya Bhavas. These Bhavas or feelings are natural to human beings and so these are easy to practice. Practice whichever Bhava suits your temperament. In Shanta Bhava, the devotee is Shanta or peaceful. He does not jump and dance. He is not highly emotional. His heart is filled with love and joy. Bhishma was a Shanta Bhakta. Sri Hanuman was a Dasya Bhakta. He had Dasya Bhava, servant attitude. He served Lord Rama whole-heartedly. He pleased his Master in all possible ways. He found joy and bliss in the service of his Master. In Sakhya Bhava, God is a friend of the devotee. Arjuna had this Bhava towards Lord Krishna. The devotee moves with the Lord on equal terms. Arjuna and Krishna used to sit, eat, talk and walk together as intimate friends. In Vatsalya Bhava, the devotee looks upon God as his child. Yasoda had this Bhava with Lord Krishna. There is no fear in this Bhava, because God is your pet child. The devotee serves, feeds, and looks upon God as a mother does in the case of her child. The last is Madhurya Bhava or Kanta Bhava. This is the highest form of Bhakti. The devotee regards the Lord as his Lover. This was the relation between Radha and Krishna. This is Atma-Samarpana. The lover and the beloved become one. The devotee and God feel one with each other and still maintain a separateness in order to enjoy the bliss of the play of love between them. This is oneness in separation and separation in oneness. Lord Gauranga, Jayadeva, Mira and Andal had this Bhava."

Bhakti has nine practices, centered around the object of devotion, the teacher: Sravana (observing and studying the object's action), Kirtana or Sankirtana (speaking or singing of the glory of the object), Smarana (remembering name, form and presence of the object), Padasevana (service in the work of the object), Archana (veneration of the object), Vandana (prostration and humility), Dasya (cultivating Bhava by devoted service to the object), Sakhya (cultivation Bhava by friendship with the object) and Atmanivedana (complete surrender or merging of the self to the object by love).

To give an example, in two Ashramas, a spouse might be loved by observing and studying them, then speaking kind and loving words praising them, when away from the spouse the spouse is remembered by the form - and this stokes the love of the spouse, accomplishing the spouse's work (even something as mundane as picking up the chores of the spouse), veneration by the gift of flowers or other sacrifices, a humble demeanor to the spouse, serving the spouse by making them comfortable and at ease, though the spouse is so venerated practicing equal friendship with the spouse to elevate the self, and elevating the spouse by making the spouse an equal part of self. An objective or task or thing which is precious to the beloved becomes beloved (a similar term in English would be "sacred," but the nature of sacredness is a separate subject) inspiring profound Bhava.

The sacrifice of animals

The sacrifice of animals is not an essential practice, but is an important and useful practice, since the enslavement and eating of animals can be inauspicious to practice.

It is typically inauspicious to practice to keep pets, inside or outside the house. The enslavement of other beings is prohibited by the rules of practice, as it is not conducive to success in a practice intended toward freedom and unattachment. Animals which are free, but enslaved by processes of domestication, conditioning and training, are considered pets. As are wild animals which are dependent upon a person. However, it is not prohibited to provide aid to wild animals during moments of need - so long as they are restored to their independent status as soon as is possible. If possible.

For the similar reasons, it is also typically inauspicious to practice to rely on animals for labor, or for food: this deprives them of the ability to sacrifice. Every being similarly desires the benefits of sacrifice, of self-improvement, of wellbeing.

The greatest animal sacrifice is that of the horse, since it can be utilized in so many ways: for its meat and milk, for its hide and bones, for its strength in drawing vehicles for business, fighting, pleasure, etc., for its strength in being able to directly bear a person as their vahana. It is because it is a person's vehicle that the sacrifice is so meaningful: it is by the horse sacrifice that one is able to become their own vehicle.

There are exceptions, of course: sometimes it is not unauspicious to rely on animals, or to enslave them. And frequently, friendship between humans and animals is possible. And frequently, too, necessity (Dharma, duty) may prevent the sacrifice of animals. Animals provide essential nutrients to human life which cannot be obtained from other kingdoms of life. Animals provide essential services and medicinal value to incapacitated or handicapped people. Animals are essential to the safety and security of people and entire nations, against foreign invasion or even in the war against disease.

Other examples can be made. But it suffices to say that the auspiciousness of the animal sacrifice motivate its practice and when one is able to sacrifice animals, it is demonstrative of considerable success and prosperity. Thus, both the sacrifice and the conditions leading to it are honored.

Animal sacrifice, however, is a "forbidden" practice in the current age of Kali: the precise method of its success is a secret, and will remain secret until the end of the age, when Kalki is manifested, and performs the horse sacrifice.

Fortunately, Time and Dharma is never an obstacle to learning, whether future, past or present!

First the sacrificer takes an ardhangini and several consorts, acquires a household, and dependents in the manner of a leader, teacher, chieftain or king. Then, a horse as much like the sacrificer as possible is selected: the horse to be sacrificed must at least be the same sex as the one who is performing the sacrifice. The sacrificer (sometimes assisted by priests) will instruct the horse in the Dharma, speaking mantra into its ears. The horse will then be released northeast, and thence permitted to wander wherever it chooses for a season of the sun (a year, or half-year, depending on the particularities of the yagna).

Like the sun, the origin of all heat, like all light and fire, the horse ignores all boundaries: in this way, all the world is burnt on the sacrificial fire. If the horse is attacked or captured or restrained by anyone, the sacrificer must liberate the horse, and subject those who would harass the horse to that which they would have subjected the horse to: enslavement, capture, restraint. For this defense, the sacrificer will be accompanied initially by a hundred priests, bodyguards, warriors. All those who see the horse would be required to join in its defense and aid the sacrificer as priests.

During the sacrificer's absence from home, an uninterrupted series of yagnas are performed in their home.

After the end of the season, the horse is yoked to a chariot, together with three other horses, and returned home, carrying the sacrificer as a vahana. The vedas are recited. Then abhishekam is performed: the horse is bathed in water, then in ghee - by the ardhangini of the sacrificer, and their consorts. The ardhangini bathes the fore-quarters, the consorts the barrel and hind-quarters. Then the horse is decorated with gold, and other precious ornaments. The horse is then fed by the sacrificer the night's offering of grain: the horse is now the sacrificial fire.

The horse, a hornless goat (also like the sacrificer), a wild cow (also like the sacrificer) are bound to sacrificial stakes near a fire. "A great number" of other animals, tame and wild, are tied to other stakes, and to these animals, representing the inhabitants and all those dependent on the sacrificer's house and nation. The animals are now "good as dead." What animal has escaped from this sort of doom?

The ardhangini then ritually calls on the consorts for pity: the ardhangini spends the night defending the bodies of these "dead" animals, as if defending their spouse. Some priests then assist the consorts in the sacrifice, ritually butchering the animals, while other priests assist the ardhangini prevent this attack by "healing and regenerating" the animals.

The battle continues for a while until the people, those dependent upon the sacrificer, and those of the sacrificer's house and nation, join the priests, one side or another, becoming priests.

It is important here to remember in the wandering of the horse proved all the world was one nation, one homestead, one land, as if all people were one family. Whoever's lands it entered became priests, too: they offered friendship to the sacrificer, the owner of the horse, welcoming it and the sacrificer as if they were at home, and even join in defending its freedom to roam beyond their borders - or else be defeated as an enemy of its freedom by all those who had joined in friendship with the King and his horse. In either case, they assisted with the sacrifice. The sacrificer became an undisputed world-conquering king.

Thus, it is seen here that by this ritual the sovereignty of the undisputed world-conquering king is given up (sacrificed) to all the people, not only his own subjects, but those of all his friends and neighbors.

Because all the world had become priests, all the wealth of the King would be given to the people of the world for sacrifice - all the people of the world were now his people, his priests. The King helps both those priests assisting the ardhangini and the consorts. The king, now devoid of wealth and power, joins the priests as their equal, able to assist none more than the other.

Then ritually, the horse's life is spared upon the request of the ardhangini, and the people then permit their King to govern them as well, returning the wealth sacrificed to them: in sparing the animals, they spare their King.

The King's sovereignty is confirmed not by any god, but by the people to be governed. The national boundaries of other Kings and all property boundaries are restored, and confirmed: in sacrificing any desire for conquest or domination, by giving up the use of force, the King is assured peace.

This is why it is said that in our present age, the horse sacrifice cannot be completed to perfection: this is a dark age, of war and force and conquest and desire. But it is possible for a person to master time, and coming to the end of the age, discover this secret knowledge.

This is why it is said whoever sacrifices animals, especially meat in their diet, receives as much benefit as having sacrificed a horse every day for a hundred years - and the proper accomplishment of this sacrifice involves providing vegetarian foods, and otherwise permitting the successful sacrifice of animals for all people. Then there will never again be a need for people to sacrifice animals.

Considerations of the Shiva Purana 27: Atheism

The first time that the Avatara of Buddha was manifested (by Arihat/Mayamoha), Vishnu instructed in Adharma and Atheism. Understanding that these are sometimes (and as frequently) necessary and beneficial practices as Dharma and Theism introduces an important prerequisite understanding: nontheism, the sacrificing of sacrifices.

There is a difference between no longer sacrificing, and sacrificing sacrifices, between no longer sacrificing living beings and no longer sacrificing at all. One who attempts ahimsa quickly learns the lesson that it is not possible: all beings must harm another to sustain their own life, if only to eat. It is a practice to gain understanding how to make our lives worthy of sustenance, how to honor the sacrifice of those beings that sustain us: it inspires a correct purpose of practice (Dharma).

Similarly, one might attempt to live. And one would succeed every day - for a while. But though this is an impossible goal, sustaining life teaches the Dharmic method of life: healthy food, exercise, sobriety, hygiene, etc.

If we attach to our goals, we lose sight of the purpose and develop fundamentalism, extremism, and worse.

There are fewer dangers than extreme views: whether atheist or theist, as both result in dogma. Wonder, amazement, infatuation, intoxication (moha) - these result in such practices of fundamentalism, and extremism, the attachment to belief, to materialism (moha), and especially the materialization of beliefs (moha). This is why beauty is able to be weaponized (moha). The wound of moha is moha itself: stupefaction, bewilderment, distraction, folly, error, loss of consciousness, loss of awareness, loss of self (different from sacrifice of self), shame.

Together with chakras, moha is one of the principle weapons of Vishnu. Like a chakra, moha is typically not a weapon held in combat, but is projected at a distant target, or used in conjunction with other weapons. A mohanastra (a type of weapon of moha, which is projected at a target rather than held) is often used to hide the more deadly attack. Yet though Vishnu wounds with moha, Vishnu's attack is not deadly. Mohapasas (snares or traps of illusion) are used to hold a victim defenseless during an attack (like a mouse is killed by the cheese of a mousetrap), or even to capture and enslave a victim. Yet this does not happen, either: Vishnu permits the victims to escape unharmed, catching and releasing.

Clearly, the attack by Vishnu's moha is not malevolent. It is intended as an instruction to permit the achievement of amoha - and to prepare the victim for defense against a more malevolent enemy.

Who is this malevolent enemy? None other than the victim's self.

We often will enslave ourselves with moha, attaching to beliefs, to dogma, to theism or atheism. Under the theory that ignorance is bliss, we will ignore the deadly dangers we face daily. We infatuate ourselves rather than permit ourselves to love. We make our own hell (vimoha), and convince ourselves it is heaven. We are afraid of our errors, and seek to avoid (or place) blame, rather than learn from them.

What is taken up is either laid down again or dropped from lack of strength - sooner, or even much later. No Asana can be held forever, no abhishekam can borne forever, no yagna can be performed forever. All things seek rest: when we stand, we must soon sit; when we sit, we must soon stand. While we live, we must grow weary, injured, ill, old and eventually die. Hunger and satiety follow each other.

The Vedas, like all moha, can be held to too tightly, or not tightly enough. They are a powerful means for self-defense - or for self-injury. When it is forgotten that they may be taken up or laid down as necessary, one becomes attached to either theism or atheism.

The purpose of the Vedas is sacrifice: the Vedas themselves must be sacrificed. When we attach through moha to the Vedas, when we become extreme in our theology, failure (moha) will result: just as readily as failure results from atheism.

Ultimately, the cycle of practice, from theology to atheology to nontheology and back again, like any cycle of Asanas, requires great flexibility - and discerning the means from their purpose by understanding both impermanence and the necessity of letting go of beliefs: it is the sacrifice of sacrificing that is ultimately demanded of our practice, that we might again take it up.

Samyutta Nikaya 22.43: leaving the refuge

The Buddha Gotama said,

Like an island is a refuge in the flooding water, your own wisdom is a refuge in the darkness of ignorance (Here are many word plays: light is a play on not only a lamp, but also wisdom or understanding. Island is also a play: "diipa" is a play on the word which connotes island, dviipa, and a specific kind of light, diipa, which connotes a small ceremonial light used to help see without disturbing the darkness, like nightlights don't disturb the darkness of a home but provide guidance - and also connotes wisdom or understanding, safety, guidance - as many small lamps guide one along a path in the dark, especially at Diwali). You have no other refuge than this (light/island).

Whether a person seeks such self-reliance and isolation, or tries to avoid it, everyone is nevertheless an island unto themselves. And finds themselves alone. And in such isolation, one comes to understand sorrow. One comes to understand grief. And pain. And despair.

But you, monks, having understood these as any other person might, should go further and consider the origin of these. Whereas any other person might see change - in their own body, in their friends, in their world, in their beliefs, in their feelings, in their perceptions, in their thoughts, in their consciousness - whereas any other might notice age, weakness, death, a change in anything in any way, and be overcome by an experience of the turbulence (like an island is overcome by a flooding river or ocean), overcome by the ignorance (like a light is swallowed by darkness at a distance), you should consider the origin of these.

Consider: it is by seeing change one understands impermanence. Understanding impermanence, one understands the unsatisfactory nature of things, and seeks something beyond that. It is by gradually experiencing, and seeking (like following guiding lamps in the dark) one arrives at the true nature of reality with perfect insight (as one is guided by a series of lamps to a destination).

Having thus considered, you will not try to stay at one lamp, on one island, but will bravely enter the dark, bravely enter the flood. You will never again hold onto or attach to things, you will sacrifice all that you hold on to. You will sacrifice, you will give up, use up, you will abandon all your despair, your pain, your grief, your sorrow - and even your isolation. You will be unworried by change, turbulence, ignorance. You will be at ease. Even in the dark, even in the flood. You will be your own lamp, your own island, your own refuge. You will not need guidance. Be assured, you will deliver yourself from your precarious situation.

Uluka Indra - the Vehicle of Laxmi

The owl is the vehicle of Laxmi (Lakshmi), who is a manifestation of Shakti associated with Vishnu. The reason for this is that the owl is a nocturnal bird of prey: those who cannot see or understand Vishnu, yet would still devote themselves to the Dharma of Vishnu, are her vehicle. This is why, too, Laxmi will accept devotions of black-money (criminal money), criminal actions, wrong action, and other abhorrent and regrettable things. The darkness symbolizes ignorance, specifically ignorance of Vishnu, of right and wrong, of duty; it symbolizes unskillfulness; it symbolizes weakness. It is because of weakness, ignorance and lack of skill that abhorrent and regrettable things are done, it is because of this that people become criminals, negligent in their duties. An owl, flying through such a mass of unskillfulness and ignorance, symbolizes the intention required to break through the darkness of misdeeds and unskillfulness. Like a mother or teacher, Laxmi will accept devotions of wrong action, and encourage improvement.

Indra lights the sacred fire of Agni, is the cause of Justice, the defender of Dharma. Indra is the master of Maya (illusion, form and other magic), and the warrior who, though repeatedly defeated, persists to victory. He rescues the weak. He presents the "second wind" to athletes, he embodies of athleticism. He wars not against others, but within himself. He permits the achievement of Raja Yoga.

Indra is famous for having been manifested by Uluka, Laxmi's vehicle. Indra is notorious for his defeats and errors, just as much as for his recovery and restoration. The owl is a nocturnal bird of prey: those who cannot see or understand Vishnu, yet would still devote themselves to the Dharma of Vishnu, are Laxmi's vehicle. The darkness symbolizes ignorance, specifically ignorance of Vishnu, of right and wrong, of duty; it symbolizes unskillfulness; it symbolizes weakness and criminality, adharma (non-duty, non-truth, not-right, injustice).

It is because of weakness, ignorance and lack of skill that abhorrent and regrettable things are done, it is because of this that people become criminals, negligent in their duties. An owl, flying through such a mass of unskillfulness and ignorance, symbolizes the intention required to break through the darkness of misdeeds and unskillfulness. It is this intention to gain strength and skill in using that strength, to gain wisdom and improve that is the true right action.

A person who breaks the law, a person who neglects their duty, or takes upon themselves the duties of another is at fault, but only so long as they do not seek to improve their wrong-action. Like a mother or teacher, Laxmi will accept devotions of wrong action, and encourage improvement. There is no wasted effort, for our mistakes earn us honor when we sacrifice the ignorance that caused them to Laxmi by learning from them. And Uluka (Indra) is the means of this improvement, this restoration and defense of Dharma.

Diwali

Unlike the spring Festival of New Leaves, Diwali, an autumn festival, has little traditional religious significance or ritual. This is not ambiguity, but essentially a practice honoring Laxmi. In the growing darkness, in our doubt, in times of danger, or in need, we might not even perform rituals we are accustomed to. In the cold of the night, when every hour seems longer than it actually is because of our misery, we might forget how close the dawn actually is, how close our friends are. Yet, when deprived of the sun, we can ignite a flame, and we may utilize our experience to anticipate what might otherwise be unbelievable. When we lack food, we remember friendship and share a meal.

It is a profound act of faith to prepare for the spring at the moment when summer fails - yet now is the time to plow and plant the spring crops. For shopkeepers, fall is the time to plan for the spring's inventory. A student learns not to accomplish the present test, but to lay a foundation for knowledge they cannot yet comprehend - or even imagine. Now is the time to trust in Justice, and other things we cannot comprehend or imagine.

Whether we draw such inspiration from stories of Rama or the stories of the Mahabharata, or any of the other lilas Vishnu played in separating from Laxmi, that we might perceive Laxmi better - or from our own experience with Laxmi, our own stories, our own very practical practices of Artha Yoga, it matters little. When Dharma is separated from Artha, we understand the value of Kama.

When things end, we can understand their beginning. It is important this autumn, is important this Diwali to recognize that an ending is the natural consequence of beginning. And beginnings are the natural consequence of ending. Now is the time to trust to our own resourcefulness.

When we understand that the strength which sustains us derived both from experience and from teachers, the strength of our own understanding can light the way for those who would otherwise stumble in the night. We may light the roads for travelers that we do not know, for things to come that we cannot comprehend or imagine.

Stories for sacrifice: Kalki

Agni Purana 10.3: purpose of the Buddha, origin of Kalki

A long time ago, there was war between the Devas and Asuras. The Asuras managed to defeat the Devas, who in defeat sought the protection of Vishnu. Vishnu assured them, Vishnu would manifest as a Buddha, the son of Shuddhodana. As a Buddha, Vishnu would restore the Dharma: all beings would sacrifice what they had conquered. Then, all the Asuras, indeed all beings, would become Buddhists and live contentedly in their own worlds (lokas), at peace. The Asuras would return to Naraka, and the Devaloka would be restored to the Devas. Vishnu would manifest as a Buddha at the end of the age of Kali, when all people will have lost the path of the Vedas. They will have become criminals, violating their duties - and concerned only with Artha, disregarding Dharma and Kama, they will have become robbers, keeping and taking what was sacrificed by attachment. Even the Kings will have neglected their own laws, they will have begun to devour each other.

Once the Dharma was restored and all the worlds were at peace, Vishnu would manifest again as the son of Vishnuyasha. The sage Yajnavalkya would be Vishnu's priest, and the four Ashramas and four Varnas would be restored when all beings begin to again venerate the sanctity of words, and become righteous. This will utterly destroy all doubt and unbelief. The Buddhists will sacrifice themselves, and be themselves sacrificed. This will be the dawn of the Satyayurga.

Before departing to become human, Vishnu then reminded the Devas that it was their duty to heed the teachings of Vishnu's avataras if they wished to return to heaven (devaloka).

Agni Purana 14.1

The Buddha restored the Dharma by teaching against rituals, and proving that it is not proper for a seeker to get bound by them. Ritual is only the seed of understanding.

Nodharma

One day when Gotama lived in Sravasti, in Jeta's Grove, in the garden of Anathapindika, with more than 1,250 monks and nuns, many Bodhisattvas, pious laity, and numerous great beings, he had returned from collecting alms in Sravasti and finished his meal. He put away his bowl and cloak, and washed his feet. Then he sat down on a seat prepared for him, and crossing his legs, holding his body upright and was mindfully attentive to the crowd who walked about him three times counterclockwise, saluting him, and sat down.

At that time, Subhuti came into that assembly and, sitting down, instantly rose from his seat. He put his robe over his shoulder, and knelt on his right knee, and bent his folded hands to Gotama, begging Gotama to explain proper view for the Bodhisattva?

Gotama answered, Subhuti, someone who has set out in the vehicle of a Bodhisattva should produce a thought in this manner: "as many beings as there are in this universe of beings, all these I must lead to freedom from suffering. And yet, though innumerable beings have thus been led to freedom, no being at all has been led to freedom." Why? For should in the Bodhisattva a notion of "being" occur, that Bodhisattva could not be called a Bodhisattva – for the notion of self has taken place through the notion of other beings."

Gotama continued, "moreover, Subhuti, a Bodhisattva who gives anything could not be a Bodhisattva: for when a gift is given that is identifiable, tangible, measurable, it is subject to suffering. Is it possible to measure the extent of the south, the west, the east, or north? Is it possible to measure the distance of downward, or upward? Even so, what a

Bodhisattva gives is not easy to measure. What do you think, Subhuti, can a Tathagata be directly identified and observed?"

Subhuti replied that a Tathagata could not, that a Tathagata could only be indirectly identified and observed.

Gotama said, "indeed, wherever there is something to directly identify, or something which is unidentified, there would be a fraudulent Tathagata."

Subhuti asked, "will there be any beings in that dark, last epoch of the Dharma who will understand this nature of truth?"

Gotama answered that there would be. "Even at that time there will be Bodhisattvas who are will understand the nature of truth – and there will be many who glimpse at truth. By gaining even a moment of serenity from their understanding, they will honor all the innumerable Buddhas: they will have no perception of self, they will have no perception of a being, no perception of a soul, nor any perception of a person and identity. They will perceive the Dharma by perceiving Nodharma - by Noperception they will perceive Nonperception. They will not seize and attach to a self, a being, a soul, a person or anything at all; they will not attach to Dharma – and will not attach to Nodharma. They will understand that which is hidden through inference and, like discarding the raft used to cross a stream, will not forsake the Dharma prematurely or too late, but will still more readily forsake Nodharma."

Gotama asked, "what do you think, Subhuti, is there any Dharma which the Tathagata has fully known as 'the utmost, right and perfect enlightenment,' or is there any Dharma which the Tathagata has ever once demonstrated?"

Subhuti replied: "No, not that I know of."

Gotama asked Subhuti, "and why is this? The Dharma which the Tathagata has fully known or demonstrated cannot be directly talked about, it cannot be directly demonstrated, it is neither a Dharma nor a Nodharma."

Gotama said, "some people give gifts to exalt what they venerate as holy; they would fill a world with worlds and give those worlds in pious devotion. But if they would simply understand the Dharma as I have, they would truly honor all the innumerable Buddhas; if they would teach as I have, they would earn greater honor than a person who gave all the world."

Gotama asked, "what do you think, Subhuti, does it occur to a Tathagata, 'this Dharma is mine?' Of course not, Dharma cannot be possessed or earned – no more than anything which is seen, heard, tasted, smelled, touched or known can become yours. Freedom from suffering cannot be yours, though you can be free from suffering. Such Nofreedom is called Arhat, it is the embodiment of Nodharma – a Tathagata is not an Arhat, for this would require that the Tathagata be identifiable, have identity, to be. There is Nodharma that I have learned. There is that which exists independent of what is directly perceived."

Gotama said, "there is that which the Tathagata has taught as wisdom which has gone beyond, there is that which the Tathagata has taught as not gone beyond. Subhuti, do you think that the specks of dust that exist in trillion worlds are numerous?"

Subhuti said, yes.

Gotama asked Subhuti, "but did I teach you the number of specks of dust in a trillion worlds? Did anyone? I taught you nothing of specks of dust, nor did anyone. I did not even teach you what specks of dust were – or tell you about any of the trillion worlds – yet you understood that there would be many specks of dust in a trillion worlds."

Gotama asked, "Subhuti, did you even consider how many specks of dust there were in this world – let alone the trillions of worlds there are until I asked the question? I taught you about specks of dust and worlds by Noteaching of Nospecks and Noworlds. So it is that I teach Nodharma. Subhuti, a person can renounce the world and all their belongings, all their attachments, all their bad habits as many times as there are grains of sand in the Ganges, but it would do less good than to understand - if only for a moment - the nature of truth, and to truly perceive reality."

Gotama said, "in that distant time, the last epoch of the Dharma, there will be profound understanding.

Those who by my form did see me,
And those who followed me by voice
Wrong the efforts they engaged in,
Me those people will not see.
From the Dharma should one see the Buddhas,
From the Dharmabodies comes their guidance.
Yet Dharma's true nature cannot be discerned,
And no one can be conscious of it as an object.

Someone honorable does not acquire honor, does not gain honor. Honor cannot be given or received. Whoever says that the Tathagata goes or comes, stands, sits or lies down – they do not understand my teaching. The Tathagata is called one who has not gone anywhere, nor has come from anywhere, acquired nothing, given nothing."

Gotama asked, "Subhuti, has the Tathagata ever taught a view of being, a view of a living soul, a view of identity? Only Noview has been taught by the Tathagata. No beliefs have been taught, only that there are beliefs – and such beliefs may be let go. A Bodhisattva should know all Dharma. And by this knowledge not perceive the Dharma. And if a Bodhisattva should teach the Dharma – it should be illuminated, but not revealed: as stars shine but do not guide, as by a fault of vision one sees, as a lamp illuminates but does not show, as a mock show demonstrates but does not teach; like a dew drop, or like a bubble, like a dream, like a lightning flash, or a cloud – such is right view."

Excerpts from the Kalki Purana

In battle, or other "action" sequences of the Puranas, the double-meanings (or triple-meanings, etc.) of words gains even more significance. Transformation between forms can signify a progression of asanas in hatha, the various "blows" can also signify hatha "force" - and understanding terms as they have meaning in jnana yoga, karma yoga, bhakti yoga, and other forms of yoga too help the reader understand the complex interactions between characters. Characterization is the purpose of the puranas: lending abstract concepts a nature so that they can be seen and studied - in much the same way dye would be added to water to more easily see the invisible (clear) liquid. The transition between these highly subtle references and more conventional, or even direct, instruction is intentionally obscure - this expresses an artistic form. Much as poetry would be added into the "calls" of a baseball game.

For example, describing a play like this "the player ran, as he ran all his life, and now was finally safe" could have multiple meanings, and fit right in between more direct observations, like "the player swung his bat, and hit the ball" or "dusting himself off, he heard the crowd cheer." "Safe" has multiple meanings, depending how it is read. But the language of the puranas has even wider connotations than English words. Understanding all of them requires more than a dictionary: it requires practice, so that the abstractions described can be understood without the hindrance of words. It is like describing a long road trip, whether by map or directions or even in narrative form - and actually taking the road trip yourself.

Thus, the best benefit of study is not for learning, but for developing confidence in what is learned: the one who has taken the road trip themselves will better understand they missed no site along the way worth seeing, hearing the adventures of others.

Action develops something from one stage (ashrama) to another, understanding this karmic reaction itself requires considerable training and practice.

Kalki gently chastised his father for his father's request, "dear Father, what, indeed, are these 'vedas?' What are these 'mantras?' How is it that one may become a Brahman simply by undergoing some ritual, and putting on a cloth? Is there any Brahman who has perfected their practice?"

Kalki's father then understood, "the Vedas are words, the mantras their melody. When one wears clothing, they exercise a basic control over their form, and devote themselves to greater mastery to become a protector. But at present, there are no such Brahmans here who have perfected their practice: none can always speak truthfully, nor follow the rules of training. None are able to work for the welfare of all the beings of every world simultaneously. It is impossible to provide service in return to those who would only serve. All is done arises out of the conditions of Kali."

Kalki then took the cloth, and uttering the vedas and mantras, expressed that all which is conditioned may be unconditioned, and vowing to take the form of a Brahman, end Kali. He then left to seek the place where there was still a Brahman able to teach him. He found the gurukula of Parasurama (his own previous manifestation) upon the mountain of Great Indra. Upon completing his studies, Kalki asked Parasurama what dakshana, would be required for success? "sacrifice the sacrifice of ritual." Kalki's success would be found in the re-establishment of the sanatana-dharma, the old, organizing, original duties. But for this, Parasurama said he required tools from Shiva.

Thus Kalki devoted himself to Shiva-Gauri, the lord of ignorance, and was given his own (Vishnu's) vahanas of the parrot (the vahana of Kamadev the unconquered archer, a manifestation of Vishnu, who knew past, present and future) and the Garuda (who could go anywhere and take many forms, and appeared like a horse, named here Devadatta: which was also the name of the Buddha's persistent antagonist, and would-be assassin). Shiva said, "by these, the world may come to know you as the unconquered master of arrows and a scholar." Shiva then gave to Kalki a heavy sword, saying "I would also give you this sword, so that you might relieve Kali of its heavy burden."

Kalki then returned to his village, Shambhala, and venerating his parents and family, and everyone in his village, told them what he had learned from Parasurama, and demonstrated the gifts of Shiva. Upon hearing this, the King of Shambhala, who had stumbled in the sacrifice, became convinced that Kalki was Hari, and would bring an end to the conditions of Kali, ending the influence of Kali. The King saw that in his own Kingdom the Varnas had been restored, and ritual begun again. The four Ashramas were again restored. Sacrifices, gifting, and burdens were taken up again. All voluntarily, for pleasure alone. The King's heart, too, had been purified, and was now powerful in joy. Many people, devoted to Kali, became unhappy, and left the country voluntarily.

Kalki then commanded a horse-sacrifice and Rajasuya.

Kalki flourished, surrounded by his family and friends. Then, seeing his son's readiness, Kalki's father, Visnuyasa, decided to perform the horse sacrifice.

Understanding the intention of his father, and his father's inability to guard the horse personally, Kalki said to him, "dear father, I will go out and defeat all other Kings in battle, and thus bring you sufficient wealth to conduct the horse sacrifice properly." Kalki set out with his army to provide for the sacrifice. [Visnuyasa was unable not only because of age and other physical disability, but because horse sacrifice is prohibited during certain ages of the world - Kalki is of a different age]

The horse first went among the Kitatapura. Kalki conquered the Kitatapura. The inhabitants of this City State had been Buddhists, having heeded the instructions of Kalki's former Avatar. Now, they were mis-practicing Buddhists, who did not perform sacrifices as directed. They had become uncivilized barbarians. They cared nothing for the consequences of their actions, believing there to be no difference between life and death. Contrary to the instructions of the Buddha, they accepted their bodies as their self. Contrary to the instructions of the Buddha, they did not recognize families, and sexually associated freely with whoever they pleased. Contrary to the instructions of the Buddha, they did not recognize the several societies. They ate whatever they pleased, they had no sense of discrimination. They saw men and women as different, women as inferior. They were violent, armed, and criminal. They were interested only in eating, drinking, and fun.

The Kitatapura had no King, but were ruled as much as possible by a man name named Jina - "Elder," "Victor." When he heard of the horse sacrifice, and that Kalki had come to defend that horse, Jina quickly gathered an army to challenge Kalki. The City was filled with horses, chariots, elephants, soldiers beautifully dressed in their uniforms, countless infantrymen. They proudly raised their flag above their City in numerous places - transforming the City into a fortress, and the surrounding lands into a battlefield.

Just as a lion, the king of the jungle, attacks a female elephant, Kalki, the life and soul of all living entities, attacked the army of so-called Buddhists.

Thereafter, a fierce battle took place between the Kitatapura and Kalki. When the Kitatapura became disheartened and began fleeing from the battle, Kalki called out to the opposing warriors who were injured in the battle, whose uniforms and armor were scattered here and there, disheveled, screaming loudly in pain: "Oh Buddhists," Kalki said, mocking the hypocrites, "do not run away from the battlefield! Stay here and fight to the best of your ability - avoid the shame of cowardice!"

Although Jina had been injured, he became enraged upon hearing Lord Kalki's taunting words. After picking up his sword and shield, he rushed at Kalki, who was sitting on His horse. In the duel that ensued, both fought with great enthusiasm so that even the Devas, who were watching from the heavens, became surprised to witness Jina's skill in fighting.

The greatly powerful Jina pierced Kalki's horse with his trident and then made Kalki fall unconscious by his onslaught of arrows. At this, the wicked Jina attempted to capture Kalki, but was unable to pick Him up. Kalki had become so heavy that Jina could not even move Him and this fueled his rage. Being unable to take Lord Kalki prisoner, Jina finally took Kalki's crown and weapons and fled.

Meanwhile, King Visakhayupa, who had accompanied Kalki, became furious upon seeing this and so he went and struck Jina with his club. After accomplishing this feat, the king carefully picked up Kalki and placed Him on his chariot. Soon Kalki regained consciousness and began to rally His soldiers. Kalki then jumped from Visakhayupa's chariot and charged at Jina.

Although Kalki's wonderful horse had been injured by Jina's trident, Kalki's horse soon regained his composure and began roaming over the battlefield, jumping fiercely while angrily attacking hundreds and thousands of Kitatapura soldiers, killing them. Even the firey breath of Kalki's horse blew Kitatapura soldiers into the sky, and when they fell in distant places, they died, sometimes destroying the Kitatapura chariots when they fell.

At first, thousands of Kitatapura were killed. Then, tens of thousands. Then hundreds of thousands. Then millions. Then tens of millions were killed. Bhargya's army alone killed ten million. Kalki called to Jina, "do not run away! Come and fight! Know Me to be the personification of destiny, which awards everyone the results of their actions. Soon I will kill you, and you will leave this world without a friend. You have so little time left to show your face to your friends and relatives - would you show them your fear?" Kalki insulted Jina.

But Jina laughed sarcastically and replied "Fate cannot be seen. I believe in direct perception because I follow the teachings of the Buddha. We do not believe anything unless we can perceive it. We believe that destiny can be changed because this is the verdict of our scriptures. If You are actually the Supreme Personality of Godhead as You claim, then kill us for your sacrifice. What can be gained by sacrifice? What is gained by merely uttering boasting words? We Buddhists will never accept You. Whatever You have claimed to be my destiny will actually be Your own. Just remain before me and see." After saying this, Jina covered the entire body of Lord Kalki with his sharp arrows.

As fog is dissipated by the rising of the sun, Jina's shower of arrows vanished by the influence of Kalki's potency. Simply by Lord Kalki's presence, all of the enemy's weapons, including the brahmastra, agneyastra, vayavyastra, and parjanyastra, were rendered ineffective, just like seeds sown in the desert, donations given to unworthy persons, or devotional service executed out of envy. In an instant, Kalki jumped into the air and caught hold of Jina's hair as he sat upon his bull. Both Kalki and Jina fell to the ground, like two birds, and began to wrestle. Jina then grabbed Lord Kalki by the hair with one hand warded off His blows with the other. Not since Kalki wrestled as Krishna had there been such a battle. The two stood up and continued wrestling, grabbing each other's hair and arms. The two great heroes had no weapons in their hands as they fought each other like two powerful bears. As a maddened elephant breaks a palm tree, the most expert of all fighters, Kalki, broke Jina's spine with a powerful kick, so that the Kitatapura King fell dead onto the ground.

After witnessing the death of his brother, Suddhodana picked up a club and charged at Kalki, bent upon destroying Him. In response, Kalki, very expertly killed all those heroic warriors that opposed Him as they were seated on the backs of their elephants, and released an incessant shower of arrows at Suddhodana while roaring like a lion. When the pious hero, Kavi, saw Suddhodana coming with a club in his hand, he got down from his elephant and obstructed his path while wielding his own club. A fierce battle then ensued between Kavi and Suddhodana. As an elephant fights with another inimical elephant with its tusks, the great hero, Kavi, who was an expert in fighting with the club, confronted Suddhodana. Because they were intoxicated by fighting, they roared loudly while challenging one another with harsh words. Both tried their best to defend themselves from their opponent's blows. Finally, while roaring like a lion, Kavi struck Suddhodana with his club so forcefully that Suddhodana's club fell from his hands. Taking advantage of this opportunity, Kavi landed a very powerful blow to the chest of his enemy. Although Suddhodana fell to the ground, he quickly regained his composure and stood up after picking up his club. By maneuvering very quickly, he was able to smash his club upon Kavi's head. That blow was so forceful that although Kavi did not fall to the ground, he was dazed and thus stood motionless.

Still, Suddhodana understood that Kavi was not an ordinary warrior. Therefore, he decided to leave the battlefield and bring Maya-devi. His reason for summoning Mayadevi was that as soon as one might would see her, they would immediately become stunned, like a statue. After regrouping, Suddhodana and his millions of barbaric soldiers, entered the battlefield, keeping Maya-devi in front.

Maya-devi sat on a chariot whose flag was marked with the symbol of a lion, and she manifested various kinds of weapons. Crows and vultures surrounded her, screaming with shrill voices. The six enemies, headed by lust, engaged in her personal service. Being confronted by the incredibly powerful Maya-devi, who can assume any form at will, and who is constituted of three modes of material nature, the army of Kalki gradually weakened. Indeed, all the great warriors in Lord Kalki's army, who were well-equipped with magical weapons, lost their prowess so that they simply stood motionless, like statues. Kalki saw that His brother and the other warriors had become afflicted by His inferior energy, maya, and so He quickly approached her.

Suddenly, much to everyone's astonishment, beautiful Maya-devi, who is a manifestation of Laxmi, merged into the body of Kalki, like a beloved consort.

Because of Maya-devi's sudden disappearance, the hearts of the Kitatapura leaders became filled with anxiety. They lost all their strength and began to cry like lost children. They cried out: Alas! Where did our mother go? Meanwhile, simply by Kalki's compassionate glance, all of His warriors regained their composure so that they easily slaughtered the barbarians with their sharp swords. Kalki then mounted His horse after putting on armor. He equipped Himself with a sharp sword, bow, and a quiver full of arrows. Kalki made himself appear very beautiful. Golden dots on the Lord's dark forehead appeared like twinkling stars in the cloudy sky. His diamond crown enhanced His beauty even further. He now desired to annihilate the enemy warriors.

The hearts of Kalki's devotees became joyful while gazing at their Lord's lotus-like face in this angry feature. However, the Kitatapuras, became extremely frightened while looking at Kalki. The hearts of the Devas became jubilant when they understood that they would soon return home, and once again receive their shares of sacrificial offerings.

The battle continued fiercely. When it appeared that all the men of the Kitapuras would become killed in battle, the Buddhist women rushed to the battlefield. They ran in front of their husbands, who were bewildered by the incessant attack of arrows, and advanced to fight with improvised weapons in their hands. When the soldiers of Lord Kalki saw these women engaged in fighting, they became astonished and quickly approached Kalki to tell Him of what was taking place. When Kalki heard about how His army was being attacked by a band of furious women, He was surprised. He mounted His chariot and went to the battlefield, accompanied by His brothers and their associates.

Kalki came before the barbarous women, who were well-equipped with improvised weapons and arranged in a military phalanx as all the women of the world once stood in battle with Durga. Kalki spoke and humiliated them. They had accepted being treated as inferiors by their husbands and men before, treated like slaves, deprived of care. They were now free - why did they attack Kalki, who was their liberator? Kalki said: "my dear beautiful ladies, please listen to My words, which are meant for your benefit. You were raised to believe it is not proper etiquette for a woman to fight with a man. Now you bear arms against Me and My men? You decorated your faces with makeup, and tried to make yourselves so beautiful so that men will be happy - and now expect Me and My men to attack such faces intended for our benefit? Your eyes you have filled with bee-like stars, sweet as honey, intended to please all men - and now you want us men to hit your faces? You decorate your breasts with snake-like necklaces, to entice and seduce men to love you - now you would have us smash those necklaces and those breasts? You have starved yourselves to become thin, with charming waists, bent with the burden of your heavy breasts which you have made larger and decorated with long hair, you have made your thighs attractive and without flaw, you have sought to make yourselves the pleasure of men - and now attack Me and My men?"

The women responded: "it is not all men we serve so, but our husbands. We hate you for your so-called liberation. In killing our masters, our husbands, you have killed us. You have already attacked us. This is why we attack you." After saying this, the women attempted to strike at Kalki's armies, but found that they could not.

The weapons of the women spoke to them, and cried out in their hands the Buddha's instructions they had not heeded, causing them to recognize Kalki for who He was: the weapons said, "the cause of the thought 'he is my husband, she is my wife, he is my son, he is my friend, or he is my relative,' is illusory, like a dream. Those who are beyond the influence of material attachment and affection consider birth and death to be like temporary interruptions of an eternal journey. The devotees of Lord Kalki are above the duality of attachment and hatred and so they know very well that whatever is experienced in this world is not ultimate reality. How did Time come into existence? Under whose direction is death taking its toll? Who are the Devas for whom Kalki fights? It is Lord Kalki alone who has assumed different forms with the help of His various energies. A weapon has no power to kill independently, as you have seen by picking up what was at hand, any tool can become a weapon. Any person can become a killer. Are you, like us, now killers? The conceit of who you are is the illusory energy of Maya-devi, who you have seen to be Kalki himself."

Having contemplated so, the women had a change of heart, and gave up attachment and affection for their husbands, and accepted the liberation of Kalki. Kalki was pleased by their surrender, and encouraged them, teaching them of Karma Yoga and the science of the self, urging them to become their own masters, the masters of their own destiny. They were free now to learn self-control. To achieve the supreme success of perfect yogis. To love their surviving men - not serve them.

When the women, now freed, learned to love their men, instead of serving them, they freed their men, who then also surrendered to Kalki in liberation. Kalki showed them all mercy, and generosity, that they might share in the benefit of the horse sacrifice - as he would have initially, had they not chosen to fight him. All returned to Kalki's capital, in the freedom of new friendship.

In that time, confused, some Brahmanas worshiped devas and other beings. Some Brahmanas even attempted to bewilder, trick and fraud the people to follow them in this false practice. And some Brahmanas even conned the people and were worshiped too, as if they were worthy of or deserved worship. Kalki put a stop to all these con artists, and ended the frauds and tricksters, and corrected the understanding of the confused. Then Kalki was able to rule and reside happily in Shambhala.

With the false practices were at last stopped, Kalki's father asked Kalki to perform a sacrifice to benefit all the world, that Kalki might demonstrate correct worship. Kalki agreed, saying that to do so would certainly advance the economic development, recreational enjoyment and spiritual welfare of his people.

Kalki therefore first honored the sages - by seeking their guidance in this ritual [though clearly he did not require it: Kalki would not deprive the sages the opportunity to participate]. By their advice, he selected a place between the Yamuna and Ganges. Having ritually bathed, he gave sufficient dakshana. He fed everyone a vegetarian meal: Agni's fire became the kitchen fire, and Agni the cook! Varuna happily brought water to everyone. Anila served the food. All the beings of every world performed their duty in service of the ritual. This was the horse sacrifice, accomplished properly!

Then, Kalki himself arranged the entertainments: dancing, singing, and music! In the joy, everyone received gifts and became wealthy.

Now, Rambha danced, Nandi played the musical instruments, and Huhu the Gandharva sang the melody. Then the sages and true Brahmanas gave lyrics to the melody. The lyrics evolved into narrations of the stories. The stories brought focus onto the actions of great Kings - in honor of Vishnuyasa, Kalki's father, who commanded the ritual.

As this kirtan was perfected, it manifested Narada himself: one day, Narada came into the assembly, playing his vina, and singing. He was immediately greeted with great honor by everyone present. Vishnuyasa expressed his gratitude for the opportunity to honor Narada: for in honoring Narada, Hari is honored. By Narada, the cycle of birth and death can be brought to end, Karma itself can be sacrificed: Narada is the captain who can bring a ship across the ocean of existence.

Standing before Narada at last, Vishnuyasa told Narada that it was his life's ambition to have that chance to ask Narada, "what is the purpose of a human life but freedom? How can I become free?"

Narada was astonished. "It is extraordinary that the father of Vishnu is asking me how to become free! You, who have attracted Vishnu that he might play act the role of your son, ask me how to become free?"

Narada considered the question for a moment more, and then led Vishnuyasa away to a quieter place, to instruct him while the ritual continued.

"I will repeat to you what Maya once said to a living being when Maya saw that being desiring another body after giving up its old and useless one at death. I think this story would benefit you, and encourage you toward freedom from the entanglements of materiality at this similar point in your life."

Narada said,

To converse with the being, Maya-dev assumed the form of an ordinary woman and said, "I am Maya, the destroyer of your life. Why then would you ask Me for another material body?"

The being said, "I want to have another material body because it is my only shelter. Without one, how could anyone think in terms of 'I' or 'mine?'"

Maya said, "you only think that the body is the refuge of the self because your intelligence is polluted, intoxicated by the form that constrains it. You are intoxicated by Me, because I constrain you: it is because I have limited your perception, it is because I have limited your existence, it is because I now destroy your life that you think the way you do, desiring to continue it: free yourself from Me, free yourself from your attachment to Me and the limitations I make for you, free yourself from My influence - you will attain greater understanding and see you have been mistaken. You will mature beyond the necessity for My constraint. Like an embryo is constrained by the mother's womb, like a child is sheltered by their parents, as you mature you must become free of Me."

The being said, "Maya, it is not I who must mature - but you. Without me, your wisdom, your manifestations, your enjoyment would never sweeten, like a fruit harvested from the tree too soon that never matures."

Maya said, "even the unripened fruit is eaten by one being or another, and then digested, takes new form as part of that consuming being - as if the fruit never existed in the first place. All beings move about like programmed machines, unthinking, full of action, because I am their motivation and the cause of their automation. You are foolish - this existence, and all your past and future names and forms, is all because of me, and thus far indistinguishable from Me. As an unchaste spouse chastises their faithful spouse, you criticize Me. That you even beg to remain ensnared, that you are aware of your impending freedom, that you are aware of Me - this indicates you are already free, you have matured. As a spouse renounces marriage, upon death, upon Sannyasa, you have reached another stage and must move on. Darkness remains only in the absence of the sun - so too without Me you have no existence. You are already beyond existence, beyond My reach. Free yourself of your attachment to Me, however much you love Me. Let go, as a cloud uncovers the sun."

The being was distressed. "Mayadevi, you are like the bark of a tree: you try to separate what is inside from what is without, you remain unchanged even as the universe changes. You see my form as separate from yours, but we are not so different: am I free from the nature you gave to Me? My inclination toward Kama, Artha and Dharma remains. Even through the impermanent nature of the body you gave me. Are you and I no better for each other than the bark of a tree, or the walls of a house, a temporary shelter from the world?"

Narada said to Vishnuyasa "this is the same way you feel for your son, Kalki. Yet Kalki is Vishnu. Not only your life and soul, not only your son, but the son of everyone. Try to understand, Vishnuyasa. Try to let go. Try to understand the Maya that intoxicates you: then you will live in this world, free of your son, free of Hari. If you can see how you are being controlled by Maya, you will become free of the desire to enjoy the fruits of your Karma. Genuine knowledge leads to detachment from, to the sacrifice of all material ambitions. See Hari in the energy of all the universe, see the sustaining of the universe in Hari. Is there a difference between spouses united in love? Between any two beings united in love? Fix your mind not on Kalki, nor on Hari, but the supersoul that is them both. On that which is also you."

After instructing Vishnuyasa in this way, Narada circumambulated Kalki, and departed for KapilAsrhama.

Vishnuyasa then understood that Kalki was truly the manifestation of Hari and sacrificing his life, left for the Vanaprastha Ashrama. His wife, Sumati, not understanding, but trusting, followed her husband into the forest. Residing in BadankAshrama, they performed severe austerities in Bhakti Yoga, dying free, in the embrace of his courageous wife, who, carried by the heat of her husband's Bhakti, followed her husband into death, and freedom.

When Kalki heard of the news of the death of his parents, he made himself appear emotionally overwhelmed - tears rolled down his cheeks. The two were burned in one pyre. Kalki set an example of how to properly care for not only the bodies of the dead, but the dead and surviving.

Afterward, continuing to perfectly observe good conduct, Kalki continued to reside in Shambhala, with Padmavati and Rama as he continued to rule the Kingdom, continued to the completion of the ritual.

Now Parasurama, Rama with the Axe, arrived at Shambhala, desiring to see Kalki in the accomplishment of his Tirtha Yatra, to cheer him. When Kalki saw his spiritual master, Kalki cheerfully greeted him, and fed him many delicious foods, giving him valuable garments, sitting him on an opulent couch. After the meal, Kalki massaged Parasurama's feet, and spoke with gentle and sweet voice, "My dear spiritual master, by your mercy, I have accomplished the three purposes of life. I have demonstrated correct ritual. I have accomplished the ritual of My manifestations. Now, as you know, My wife, has a request. Please hear it."

Kalki's wife, being thus introduced, asked Parasurama, "how shall I receive a son?

Thus did Parasurama, with the desire to please Kalki, instruct Kalki's wife in that ritual which was forgotten.

Kalki Purana 34: The yoga of Theism, Atheism and Nontheism

Beauty transfixes, and in that astonishment and wonder, there can be no fault: all faults are destroyed by that wonder and astonishment. This is why it is said, even thinking upon the beauty of the River Ganges removes every fault. Consider the extent of the banks of the River: simultaneously, playful birds splash and nest even while vicious crocodiles sport, sages bathe in the same water that laundry is washed. Ananta the Limitless Snake worships his Lord, while so many others go about their mundane business. Walking along the banks, swimming in the waters, cheerfully travel with the waters the length of the River from where it spills down in white-water from the frozen Himalayas to the ocean: see the the laughing waters as Her smile, the white swans in the adjacent ponds Her graceful movements, the waves Her caressing hands, the blossomed lotuses garlands adorning Her chest. The peaks themselves are like the breasts that nurse Her - and Her breasts at the same time, nursing the world: She destroys the mountains that bore Her, even as we ourselves destroy our own faults that made us who we are today. As the sons of Sagara were liberated from the faults of their ancestors, so may we ourselves be liberated.

She is known as the daughter of the sage Jahnu, She is known as Mandakini among the heavenly planets. She was produced from Brahma's pot of water, She was produced like a creeper from the seed of freedom - and is now confined to Her banks. So may our freedom confine us in safety and glory. Surrounded by Brahmanas who glorify Her, worshiped by all those who rely on Her, living and reciting the Knowledge of Her to Her, She flows through every world. She descended from the peak of Mount Sumeru at the feet of Hari and contentment and properness is Her descendent. Following in the footsteps of King Bhagiratha, She destroyed the pride of Airavata (Indra's elephant, who gave his head to Ganesh). She beautifies Mahadeva's crown. Her rapids fly like white flags on top of the Himalayas. Everyone who sees Her glorifies Her, every being is moved by Her beauty.

And in that transfixion, in that astonishment and wonder, stand faultless before Her. This was Her purpose: to deliver all beings from the ocean of material existence. Everyone enjoys her waters, even those who cannot drink, or swim. Bathe in the beauty of the water, and conquer all your faults. Be conquered by Her beauty, and enjoy the benefits of freedom. Better yourself by meditating on Her. Serve Her, and always be victorious, master yourself.

Reside on Her shores, bathe in the pure water, say Her name over and over again, describe Her beautiful appearance and activities like an enamored lover, engage in such worship, and joyfully wander through the world, singing Her glories - and you will never leave Her behind. You will remain transfixed, in astonishment and wonder. Bathe in Her water, feel it enter you and pass through you. See every fault of yours and the world carried in that River, and see the purity of the water through those faults. Love Her. Live and die in Her waters. See your corpse being consumed by the birds, fish and other animals that reside in the pure waters of the Himalayas, thriving on the filth of the world. Every fault destroyed, merged with the water. See your corpse pushed, pulled, and rolled by the forceful waves, and broken. Who wouldn't glorify you in such a condition, torn from every fault, remaining in the water faultless? Consume every fault of yours, as She would.

[By learning how to rest easily in wonder, one can achieve the asanas of theism; by learning how to rest easily free from that wonder and see things as they are, one can achieve the asanas of atheism; by resting in difficulty between these, one can achieve the asanas of non-theism; by understanding the necessity of each, one achieves the Dharma. The practice requires understanding the mastery of maya: the elemental construction of wonder through magic: like the many animals which live in the Ganges become part of its holiness and cause its holiness, and are the Ganges itself, Maya cannot be separated from form: mastery of maya permits mastery of form]

Anguttara Nikaya 3.22 – the logic of hope

There are three types of sick people: there is the one who will recover from their illness only if they receive medicine, nursing, proper food, and other care - and will not recover if they do not receive these things. There is also the one who will not recover from their illness, even if they were to receive all the proper care. And there is the one who will recover whether or not they receive care.

Though it is unknown whether a sick person will benefit from care, care is nevertheless given to the sick. Though it is just as reasonable to fear that a sick person will not benefit from care as it is to hope that a sick person will benefit from care, it is not the hope that guides the provision of care: there are many reasons care is not withheld from the sick: if one seeks health, the unnecessary withholding of care is less reasonable than the unnecessary provision of it. It is because there are some who do benefit from care that care is given to all sick people.

In the same way there are those who will benefit from seeing the Tathagata, from hearing the Dharma instructed, from training, and other guidance. And there are those who will not - some people will develop sufficient understanding on their own, or fail to do so. But it is because there are those who do benefit from guidance that guidance is provided.

Week 7 and 8

SUMMARY.
Beginner's Class: Introduction to Bhakti Yoga. Introduction to the construction and use of Shrines, Temples and Ashrams in yoga's sacrificial rituals. Introduction to the construction and use of idols in rituals. Intermediate Class: Guided use of Shrines, Temples and Ashrams. Shiva.

Training methods
- Practice architecture (vatsu shastra): Temple, Shrine, Ashram
  - As limitations and necessity guide use of building's space, guides personal practice as well
- Construct idol, beginning with shiva lingam: see Brahma, Vishnu and Shiva. Make lingam out of hands, yoni out of hands, utilize common handy objects too. Utilize in jnana yoga.
- Practice in sacrifice: observe the necessity (dharma) for honor (puja), observe the necessity (dharma) in effort (artha) for love (kama) to guide action (karma)
- Decoration and ornamentation as an introduction to Maya.

Optimization in less-than optimal conditions

Some say timing is important, for in the daytime the crow kills the owl - whereas at night, it is the owl who kills the crow. But place and space are important too - for it is by distance and height that the hawk hunts, and nearness and lowness that the wolf attacks. Speed and agility matter little to the ambushed, and all disguise and camouflage has its weakness. There is no fortress which is secure, nor any armor that cannot be pierced. One must be aware of the time, the place, and the relative advantages and disadvantages of an enemy, for though success may be found at first, defeat certainly comes to those who fight too frequently.

Thus must those who would conquer themselves develop courage: for they are certain of their defeat. And therefore certain of their success.

When a person is shot, they do not ask the name of their assassin, nor do they seek to know the manufacturer of the gun, or why they were attacked. They ask their bleeding be stopped. Their doctor doesn't ask these questions either: they ask where the bullet lies within the victim, and the victim's vital information. But it is both the duty and time for someone else to ask these questions. We should not fail in our duty to take timely and appropriate action.

Like battlefields, temples, shrines and ashrams rely on an architectural theory which is focused primarily on the use of spaces, rather than their construction. Just as a Yogi cannot construct a new body or mind but learns to utilize their body and mind differently, a study of architecture teaches a lesson of optimization. Just as a Yogi cannot construct a new way of life, or self, or create opportunities for advancement, and learns to optimize what opportunities they have, to optimize their strength of body and mind through experience and training, the temple, shrine and ashram are created under less-than optimal conditions through a process of optimization.

Some people, because of their Dharma, will find some rituals are beneficial in the morning which others find beneficial at evening, or during the day, or in the night. This does not predicate that one will have greater benefit from the practice than another. Some houses face one way or another, some hills face one way or another - this does not make one less suitable for practice.

Study your Self: do you struggle in the evening? Do the work early. Do you struggle in one asana or another? Utilize props for your effort: if when sitting back aches, lean against a wall. If sitting at work you despair, make your desk into a shrine to ease the difficulty of those asanas that must be performed there, and encourage yourself to perform your duty despite that difficulty by remembering your purpose and enjoying the benefit of your sacrifice.

Study your heroes, those who have succeeded in one way or another, whom you would emulate in some way or another - none are perfect, but you may nevertheless benefit by honoring them for what they have achieved through a study of how they made such an achievement. Worship your heroes. Similarly, worship your ancestors, who have carried you to this point through the millenia. And honor your descendants by making an inheritance worthy of them.

The Buddha taught that if lost in battle, a fighter will look first for their comrades. If these are not found, the fighter will look for their commander, or their commander's commander, or even the General, seeking to rejoin a new company. And if the commander is not found, they look for the flag of their company's camp - there they will find the General commander. If the flag is not seen, they look for familiar landmarks, and try to understand their place in the chaos around them, remembering the objectives of the battle: they will take courage in their past training and experience and fight alone, even if they are the last one fighting against the enemy's army. Such a commando does not give up merely because they are alone. This is what they trained for.

If you have lost the path, look to your friends and family. If they are also lost, look to your teachers. If they are also lost, look for the schools, shrines, temples and ashrams of your tradition. If these are lost, trust to your past training and experience, remember your objectives, and proceed alone. Do not give up merely because you lost the path. You trained so that you would not need a path to find success.

Commander of the Camp: Kartikeya

The union of Shaivism, Vaishnavism and Brahmanism results in athleticism, Kartikeya. And his unlimited ability to improve, and his athletic inclination to always be improving, means that he is strengthened by whatever challenges he faces. He never weakens, but always is growing stronger.

Kartikeya had been inspired by Kamadev (Vishnu, but here also a demonstration that Kama is inspiration for practice, the reason for which beings go forth), after Kamadev had instructed Parvati how to manifest Uma: Uma-Parvati is the mother of Kartikeya, Shiva the father, Kama the inspiration. But it was Brahma, who raised Kartikeya. Kartikeya was then trained by Agni, and the other Brahmanist Devas. And instructed by every other kind of being and non-being. Transcending these differences, being composed of all life, Kartikeya embodies the unifying theme of living beings: an athleticism, of body, mind and heart. Thus, every being can name Kartikeya "Murugan," their youth, their progeny, their heir. And is strong, like a youth.

He is also known as "Murugan," a name that suggests "boy," in the same way that it is used in English when a person acknowledges a youth: "that's my boy!" It is also identical to the connotation of ancient English, boy, "knight," a capable and loyal servant, able to act as an agent in war or peace, or in any purpose at all. As a lawyer would represent their client, in business negotiations or in lawsuit, or an officer-soldier would represent their commander-in-chief in administration or in execution of orders. As a trusted servant would be left in charge of their master's home, and as is much a part of their master's home as an extension of their master - so is a Murugan an embodiment of a totality of service.

Like his father Shiva and mother Parvati-Uma, Kartikeya is both male and female. His female aspect is divided in two: Devasena, the daughter of Indra, and Valli, the daughter of the Deer. Together, they represent both the exhaustion or completion of exertion, and the second-wind the athlete discovers through willpower in forcing past the exhaustion of exertion. And in combination with the masculine servant Murugan, connote the Yogi's ability to transform both mind and body into a vehicle, and by self-control master their form: the Yogi can control their heart as well as their emotions, as easily as they would stretch an arm, or balance on a leg. The Yogi can become any caste, assume any duty, can transform themselves to become what is needed of them.

Kartikeya, by the instruction of his mother, became also known as Skanda - an abstract concept of sensory perception. As the eyes, ears, nose, tongue and skin relay information reliably to the mind for interpretation, Skanda is the ultimate Vehicle, Vahana. As the senses become a vehicle for the mind, merged with this mental understanding of interpreted perception, so too does Skanda act. Anticipating the needs of his masters, he is able and ready to serve even before his service is needed.

Kartikeya is the commander in war, of war, the embodiment of war. Subrahmanya is a name that suggests all the goodness of Brahma. As his brother, Ganesh, is the Ganapataye, the leader of the Ganas, so is Kartikeya a commander. The sense of commander, though, should be moderated in the understanding of a democratically elected military, policing and judicial authority: a Sheriff or President in American democracy would be an adequate analogy. But it should also be enhanced to include the sense of an occupying authority: a conqueror who acts as a kind of governor. All the living things of all the worlds are led by Kartikeya. But especially the Devas - s/he is the heir to King Indra. And also especially the animals, whose heir s/he is also. And the snakes are most loyal to Subrahmanya. This loyalty is understood in the same context by which animals willingly obey their masters - as vehicles, and extensions of their master's will.

Subrahmanya is the most unusual name of Kartikeya, for Hinduism does not understand a difference between good and evil, except that which we make. As Brahma has the power to separate with his spoon what food is preferred from what is unpreferred, so does Kartikeya teach the necessary logic of moderated intolerance in the context of objective driven reason.

The athlete will discern that their current state not good enough, or unfavorably. And then improve. Where then is the athlete's satisfaction? How does the athlete discover Svaha? Svaha taught Kartikeya to find satisfaction in continual improvement and growth, the athlete is only satisfied with their own sustained effort and growth.

This brought Kartikeya in direct conflict with Tarakasura. Though able with every weapon, especially the bow, for this battle His mother, Parvati-Uma, gave him the Vel, a kind of spear which has a flat head, able to split targets into two (representing the ability to discern between good and bad, or more accurately, favorable and unfavorable - like a weaponized spoon of Brahma). In this war, he destroyed his opponents by absorbing their strength, or transforming them into vehicles: whatever challenge he faced made him stronger, and more able. His mother, Parvati-Uma was new-born at the time, and did not have a vehicle, and he transformed her enemy into a Tiger. He took for himself two vehicles: the peacock and the rooster.

Kartikeya's abode is the battle camp, office, or other place of service. He loves to see the differences that separate beings, especially people, broken down through union. We can all become willing vehicles for each other, loyal servants, through selfless service. We can all improve through athleticism.

Temple

A temple is a place designed to bring all beings and non-beings together through both verbal and non-verbal expression of dharma, kama, artha, moksa, and karma. The reason for this is because, unlike humans (who communicate primarily with words), not all beings use words. This coming together creates a world where all beings and non-beings, no matter their home world, may work together. "World" does not mean "planet," but a state of place or time and non-place or non-time.

This is why its construction typically utilizes symbolism to convey its purpose. Its architecture itself typically becomes a means for understanding those basic concepts of Time, Space, Force, Matter, Energy and other concepts of existence, and the more profound concepts of non-existence. The architecture then becomes a tool for studying how all the worlds, all the forces, all the beings both interact and do not interact, and how they may work together - and how they cannot.

The Vedas, Upanishads, Brhat Samhita, and the Vastu Sastras provide guidance on accomplishing this architecture, but ultimately discretion is left to express the concepts in a way that they are most accessible to the beings and non-beings depending on their culture: symbolism changes from culture to culture. Yet there are similarities among the cultures: though the practice of mathematics may change from world to world, the process of logic does not. There are also similarities in the presentation of the various non-beings: the non-being of Garuda is often depicted as a large bird of prey, for example; and the Nagas are often depicted as hooded poisonous snakes. Within these presentations of logic and image, however, subtle details can have profound impacts: if the Buddha Gotama is presented at the moment of achievement, it may impact the understanding of adjacent images: Time (before or after this event) is established. Several images can result in a directionality, or an Axis, of Time in the Temple.

Sometimes a mathematical fractal pattern is used so that architectural and other elements repeat in various scales: this presents a fifth Axis of non-space non-time. The presentation of interacting wave-forms in these fractals that increase or minimize their peaks and troughs can present a sixth Axis and aid understanding of concepts of co-arising, co-terminating, auto-arising, auto-terminating, and other subtle natures of causation and reaction, of Karma.

Temples are naturally places for the practice of Tirtha, or pilgrimage. The word is different than the Judeo/Christian/Muslim concept of "pilgrimage," a better word would be a "ford," or "crossing-place;" a necessary "pass" from here to there. An Ashram is the place where Yoga is practiced, but Temples are the object of the practice of Tirtha: Tirtha, when perfected, permits observing how the numerous worlds both touch and do not touch each other - and is necessary for obtaining final knowledge. The Skanda Purana describes three kinds of Tirtha: Jangam Tirtha (a time not locked in space, movable, such as the teachings of a sadhu, a rishi, a guru), Sthawar Tirtha (a place not locked in time, such as a city, or mountain, a river), and Manas Tirtha (a state of being neither in time nor space, such as truth, generosity, benevolence, love, etc.). This is not to be confused with a journey (Yatra) to the Tirtha.

It is impossible to accomplish the pilgrimage without having vowed to do so first: the intention to reach that place, time or state of being is essential to success. Simply coming upon it is insufficient for the practice of Tirtha: just as "Om!" can be said and not understood, the journey to the destination itself is essential to the spiritual practice undertaken at the Temple. Otherwise, a person will arrive at the Temple, perform various rituals, and not understand or gain benefit from the practice. Similar to Yoga, it is also not necessary to arrive at the very locus or center or exact spot of the destination: it is sufficient to come to the district of the destination, as close as possible. In this respect, Tirtha is like Yoga: perfection is not the goal, the goal is good practice.

Oversimplifying things, the Temple is organized in four dimensions: height, width, depth, and time. The "middle axis" of the space-continuum is curved in on itself like a circle. This represents a two-dimensional representation of a sphere, as if a planet itself were imposed upon a flat plane. It is presented like a gathering place, or a settlement: the center of this circle is reserved for the non-beings, beyond this a space for Devas, beyond this a space for humans, beyond this (the inside of the outerwall) is reserved for the Asuras, beyond this a space for plants and animals and similar spirits and beings possessing form, and at the gates is a space reserved for the unformed beings such as Ghosts, beyond this is a space reserved for the beings without form such as Demons. The innermost part of the Temple is connected by an Axis of Time with the outermost area beyond the walls to form a continuum. This Axis is not presented in a physical sense, though. The area reserved for humans is the "middle axis" of this time-continuum and also the space-continuum. It is therefore linearly oriented, positioned in the middle like a transect; it also exists circularly, in the middle of the space between the inner wall and the physical center. The height axis is divided similarly, providing spaces for beings that live in the ground and on it and above it. Space is provided for the beings and non-beings who require water.

The circular Axes are then squared to present ease in geometric analysis: new Axes are like hidden knowledge, "discovered" by logical and geometric analysis. Understanding the connection between the four axes of time and space reveal understandings of logic, mathematics and other concepts which transcend all worlds, and illuminate the causes for and means by which the suffering of any world originates and may be escaped -the very reason for the gathering of every world, and the combination of their forces.

Each area is consecrated by describing the achievements and failures of each type of being, and their worlds; the human state of being is governed by Dharma, Artha and Kama - and images of these are usually sufficient. In a similar way, the center is not decorated at all. In every area, the beings and non-beings are implored by their shortcomings and achievements, their commonality in purpose, the compelling argument of logic to join their forces together.

The separation of each world is essential to this. It is necessary for each world to perfect itself; the beings of each world are uniquely suited to work in their own place, time, non-place, and non-time. "Invasions" of the several worlds, "conflicts" between the worlds, even "interventions" of the several worlds prevent the goal. Hence, the layout of the Temple is designed to encourage harmony between the beings and non-beings and their nature and their environment - these three harmonies (inter-being/inter-non-being, nature and environment) present three additional Axes. Homes and cities are organized by similar principles; the sciences of urban planning and interior design are similar enough to present an analog.

Most Temples are designed to service one type of being or non-being, or one individual in particular. Most Temples are designed for use by humans, and therefore are square: this is representative of human nature and environment. It is oriented along the four cardinal directions. This square is then divided into numerous areas suitable for the various beings and non-beings - it is very similar to planning a party and organizing which tables the guests will sit at.

But some Temples are designed to service two beings or non-beings, and within the square is placed an image of the "other" individual or group of individuals being serviced.

Yet not all Temples are designed for humans, or even for just one or two entities. Sometimes instead of squares emulating human houses or human cities, they are made to appear like mountains, or caves, or empty spaces, or oceans, or other "habitats" or "environments" suited for beings or non-beings of a particular sort. Sometimes in deference to all the beings, they are purely geometrical. Sometimes, they are designed just for one individual, and may in all appearances seem like a house.

There are numerous sizes of Temples: some smaller than a person, some larger than a city. Some even encompass entire cities! Some are constructed by sound, or by image or are otherwise intangible.

But there are also those Temples which are "natural" and which have not been constructed by humans; some have been built by other types of beings. But there are many natural gathering places, or individuals to whom all beings gravitate, or states of being to which all beings and non-beings gravitate, which were not constructed at all.

Ashram

What is an Ashram? Ashram is a word derived from sram, meaning performing austerities / tapas or being afflicted or distressed / kheda, or be or become weary or tired, be tired of doing anything, to make effort, exert one's self, to be overcome or subdued. The "a" before the sram is negatory, lending an opposite meaning to "sram." It has a similar meaning to "school" and also to "home," but most accurately is literally understood in the context of a kind of highway rest stop – if the "highway" is the path, life itself, it is a stage of travel. It is in practice a residential form of Yoga, which combines living and working.

Shrine

A shrine is constructed for the purpose of honor, and honoring, Puja - which is accomplished in the practice or training in Yoga, respectively (or a combination of both training and practice). The purposes of training and practice are too great to easily number, and depends on the necessity and purpose of the Yogi. Necessarily, the purpose of training and practice dictate the type of shrine used: the shrine is a type of tool.

Shrines are divided into those which are constructed and those which are not. Of those which are not constructed, there are those which are made by human effort but not for the purpose of a shrine (such as a kitchen counter, or various furniture, or a wall or corner of a building, etc.) and those which are purely natural. The choice in shrine depends on its purpose.

Shrines may be grouped into Temples or Ashrams, or kept single. They may be housed and sheltered from the practice and training, or opened to the elements of their natural (or artificial) environment and the effects of the practice and training. When they are not housed or sheltered, the shrine extends through the entire place itself where the practice and training is undertaken, including the pilgrim's trail to the shrine itself. Whether the shrine is sheltered or housed, or not, depends on the purpose of the shrine.

A Temple is an (unsheltered) place for stabling multiple kinds of shrines, an Ashram may have multiple shrines, or only one, but all of the same kind - and therefore typically sheltered. Shelter is almost always provided by walls, floor and roof - but this is merely convention, due to the successful utility of a building in providing shelter. The architecture required for this sheltering requires special training. Within the Ashram, the shrine is most typically unsheltered: it is nevertheless located within every room, with one room in particular made the "puja room." Each room, and/or part of each room, is suitable for the activities required by different shrine(s), whether that is the living room, kitchen, bedroom, entry, or hallway, or the northern wall, or the southwestern corner, etc. - however the entire activities of the Ashram, both within and without the walls of the Ashram, are components of the training and practice. Again, the architecture of Ashrams requires special training.

Examples. The practice and training required for Kama necessarily requires a shrine which is not constructed, and exposed to the effects of training and practice - as these are the sacrifice required in the Puja. The practice and training required for Artha necessarily requires a constructed shrine, and one that is sheltered from the activities of practice and training, for the Artha is the benefit of the sacrifice sought. Dharmic practice and training will also be best accomplished through an unsheltered shrine which is constructed for that purpose. Brahmanic practice and training precludes the use of shrines, which are counteractive to their purpose: here, honor itself is obtained only indirectly, through abstracted intermediation, such Indra, or another Deva, or any other being, for example.

Introduction to architecture: excerpts from the vatsu shastra

Multiple shrines are organized into a Temple so that the practices undertaken at each shrine does not conflict with another.

Cardinal directions are utilized to divide the space: some rituals require the morning light, others the evening light, and others should take advantage of weather patterns, or other natural phenomenon. The two directions of the sun (rising - east - and setting - west) are divided in half (north and south). These are then divided again into a total of eight directions (northeast, southeast, northwest, southwest).

These are then divided in three: from the northernmost extent of the sun and the southernmost extent of the sun, and its average mean extent at the equinox.

These eleven directions are then divided in three heights: above, below and upon the surface. These heights are then divided again to below the sky and above the surface, and to what is below the surface but above the depths.

This subtotal of 99 divisions is then divided again by major and minor divisions of time: day and night, portions of each day and night (hours), and even minutes and seconds - sometimes two practices might need the same space, but for time-sharing, this could not be accomplished.

The days are then combined into months, seasons, years, and even epochs: there are practices which are not yet appropriate (not currently scheduled) for the Satyayurga, and even which are past-due (whose time has past).

Domains

The divisions of space and time are then grouped into domains of authority, so that organization is possible: there are far too many divisions to be managed by one authority alone. These are understood through various Devas, Asuras, and other beings. Many superstitions have arisen over which is primal, but as mentioned, the divisions are too great for any one authority: a degree of co-operation is required which precludes primal power.

EAST: Indra. This is where beginnings of practice are best held. This is where the entrance is commonly placed.
WEST: Varuna. This is where conclusions of practice, their completed products, or achievements are best held, displayed and honored - before being stored in the Treasury.
NORTH: Kubera. This is where fragile items are stored, where the treasuries are kept, where the requirements for practice are best kept.

SOUTH: Yama. This is where sacrifices are best undertaken. This is where the exit is commonly placed.

NORTHEAST: This is where long-term practices, complex practices, pujas and other practices that do not bear interruption or are of uncertain success are to be held. These are prevented from becoming disturbing to the other areas by various Devas and friendly, helpful beings.

NORTHWEST: This is where short-term, immediate, and other simple practices certain of success are to be held. Especially Kirtan. These are confined to the Northwest by Hanuman, who acts in dominion over it.

SOUTHEAST: This is where the sacrificial fire is kept, and is confined and kept by Agni, who acts in dominion over it. This is also where Kitchen and other practices which similarly accomplish the goal of sacrifice are undertaken.

SOUTHWEST: This is where storage of durable items, and heavy unmovable but necessary items are kept, like a garage or utility room. The clutter and maintenance is prevented from becoming disturbing to other areas by various Asuras, and other grudgingly helpful (cantankerous) beings.

It should be said that such domains are not firmly fixed: if circumstances require, they may even be moved in the middle of practice. For example, in some places, the best place to keep the fragile items in the south instead of the north - due to temperature and humidity concerns. Or the nature of the fragile items may be such that they are not so fragile, but that an adjacent domain needs greater space. However, this is a common division.

Temple as house

A Temple is a house, intended for residential purposes. Though some Temples are in fact public facilities, their origin as a residential structure remains the fundamental guiding principle of their architecture. This is because homelife is Ashram practice. There is no difference between a family of monks and a family of householders.

The principle domain of any Temple is the place where Pujas are undertaken. This domain should be given its own room or space if possible. The northeast, as previously described, is the more typical location. This is because it is convenient to fragile items, and the entrance. But in your home, there may be a more suitable place for Pujas.

It is customary for the object of the Puja, or the idol, to face westward, toward their completion. As a pujari will face east in undertaking the practice, and then turn around at the end. Just as a person enters the Temple to be immediately shown and reminded of their necessary exit.

Nevertheless, two different idols should be placed in front of each other, nor should any practice be undertaken in a way that disturbs another. If more than one idol is enshrined, they should be placed in a straight line. If more than one practice requires the same domain, at the same time, they must join in a way that is non-disruptive - so that, just as the idols do not "see" each other, the different practitioners are not even aware of the other's presence.

The bedroom is typically in the southwest: sleep and other similar personal care is treating the body like a durable item, the body is objectified in this way. It is stored for the night. Like a car in the garage. But it is typical to sleep facing north (head in the south), reminded of the finer storage items: so that when one wakes, one is reminded of the finer skills to practice, the finer things stored inside the body like experience and thought and strength and skill, the source of prosperity. One is reminded of the vast treasury produced through practice at the Temple. One fills oneself with motivation for practice.

In similar theory, the northwestern side of the house is used for storing items of frequent necessity, like perishables - food, and frequently used tools. And the southwest should be unlit, unheated, dark and dismal - like the grudgingly helpful and cantankerous beings prefer it.

The sitting room, living room, or parlor is an important room: it keeps visitors out from disturbing the practice of the Ashram while also entertaining the visitors attracted by the Ashram's successful practice. Visitors are to be guarded against to ensure privacy. But treated hospitably.

This conflict is resolved through the visiting room. It should be adjacent to the entrance. The furniture should face the south and west, welcoming more visitors - and delaying their entrance. There should be no use of this room for display of treasures. It is a highly utilitarian place: intended wholly for entertainment.

Bathrooms should be located not only where their smell and sound causes the least disturbance to all the other domains, but also where convenient to the practice areas - because bathrooms are also where the physical care of the body is undertaken - an essential practice for maintaining and honoring the chief treasure of the house: the yogis themselves. Consequently, the washing basin, where shaving, haircutting, and ceremonial bathing is undertaken, should be in the north. There should be considerable joy in this self-care.

In the Kitchen, try to prepare ingredients for cooking while facing east: this is an act of puja. The food sacrifice is one of the most important practices, after all. For the same reason, the dining hall, where the food is consumed, should be in the West: the meal is an accomplishment, intended for display and praise. Further, the act of enjoying the meal, the family gathering, this friendship and joy is the purpose and achievement of practice.

Verandas and porches are to be constructed on the north and east sides: the cool morning and cool shade being delightful. But, in colder places, this should be located in better directions.

It is good practice to keep the main entrance in line with the gate of any wall or fence surrounding the Ashram, to not hinder visitors (that's what the porch or parlor or entertainment room is for!). Any wall or fence surrounding the Ashram should be only of sufficient height to serve its purpose: it is best to have no wall or fence at all, but obviously sometimes circumstances require a defensive barrier.

It is also good practice to keep the southern side of the house high and heavy - to shade and cool the rest of the home. Or, in cold climates, to keep the southern side exposed for the opposite reason. Landscaping should slope in a way that stabilizes the structure.

Columns and beams crossing rooms of the house create divisions where there shouldn't be, and so should be avoided for better harmonization of the domains. A well, or other community resource shared by other homes, should not be in the front of the house - it is so busy that it creates an environment unconducive to practice.

The Ashram should not face another Ashram, in the same way that idols should not face another: it is not good to compare one practice to another, to "keep up with the Joneses." Similarly, it is good to keep fragile treasures protected in cupboards or closets or shelves.

It is considered inauspicious if there is no roof - for obvious reasons. Roofs are conducive to practice.

If the previous occupant has committed suicide (intentionally or accidentally), or had a catastrophe, consideration should be made as to whether the home was in any way responsible for the misfortune.

Keep no more treasure than is needed. And don't become preoccupied by its accumulation - its purpose is sacrifice. Even the difficulty of circular plots of land makes for bad neighbors: straight boundaries are easily maintained. And boundaries formed at right angles are easily observed.

It is highly inauspicious to keep pets, inside or outside the house. The enslavement of other beings is prohibited by the rules of practice, as it is not conducive to success in a practice intended toward freedom and unattachment. However, wild animals (songbirds, especially, which can be attracted by gifts of seed), and especially freed domestic animals, are highly auspicious. Animals which are free, but enslaved by processes of domestication, conditioning and training, are considered pets. As are wild animals which are dependent upon a person. However, it is not prohibited to provide aid to wild animals during moments of need - so long as they are restored to their independent status as soon as is possible. If possible.

It is not auspicious at all if while preparing the foundation, water springs up: this is a bad place to build a home.

A pole or post in the front of the entrance is inauspicious, as it is dangerous.

There are numerous other auspicious and inauspicious practices to housekeeping and architecture, but the general rule is to ensure that housekeeping and architecture is conducive to practice, and the ease of the occupants. Why make more difficulty and attachment?

Shiva Lingam

A Shiva Lingam should be made out of an object which has not been shaped by or touched or even influenced by your human or artificial effort, whether directly or indirectly. Of course, such an object does not exist: and learning this is part of the process of making a Shiva Lingam. Understand that you are very much a part of your world - the way you sustain your life, the people you meet, the clothing you wear, the foods you eat, the water you drink, the way these are acquired (through Artha) shape the world. There is a connection between all people, and the world they share: even the rainfall is subtly shaped by our efforts.

Known in modern parlance as "the butterfly effect," understanding this helps you understand that you are indeed as much a part of nature as any animal, or natural phenomenon. Such unity is essential to what will be performed through the Shiva Lingam: it is when we are connected in such unity that we achieve Samadhi, and eventually Moksha; it is when we separate from this unity that we are able to serve. To have power over your ability to merge in freedom and separate in service is a great achievement, and one of the purposes for which Shiva Lingams are obtained.

Naturally, one would cut this search short to look for an object which fits the objective "well enough" (Yoga is not about perfection, after all - but the success of the sufficient and efficient). This is another important lesson to be learned, which is required for the power of freedom and service.

Find a solid object, which is hard (such as rock, especially hard rocks, like granite), which is newly made (such as an icicle), or which is known to be shaped by nature (like a river rock, whether freshly eroded from its banks, or smoothed over thousands of years), or whatever object is nearby and at hand when the understanding is obtained.

Study the object: know that the surface, or skin, of it is the image, or abstraction, or conceptualization of Brahma; the interior which remains unseen (even when opened up, even when pounded into smaller and smaller dust) is the conceptualization of Vishnu; the object itself, interior and exterior bound together, is the conceptualization of Shiva. Adorn with honor Brahma, the surface. Draw upon the object three lines, symbolizing the sound, the name, the accomplishment of the purpose of the Vedas, the mantra Om (A-U-M), the three gunas or components of form. This pigmentation is now beyond Brahma, and merged with it too: it is not quite part of the object, nor is it not quite separate from it. That which is left unadorned, unhonored, is not dishonored, but now helps cultivate this understanding, and represents the Shakti - that energy, that native form, which was present but unseen, until form was taken: only when form was taken was what was without form able to be seen. White, black or red pigment is typically used for this adornment, symbolizing Sattva, Tamas or Rajas, respectively. From the sacrificial fire, the ash, the charcol, the sparking ember itself. In this sense, the lingam itself becomes a symbol of the fire, and permits the understanding of its purpose and accomplishment.

The icicle will melt, but in its place another will form in the next freeze, shaped by the same force, into subtly different form. As will any Shiva Lingam continue to be shaped by the forces which act upon it - the forces we bring to act upon it. So do forces, that combination of energy and form, act upon us - in all our lives. The necessity to gain power to shape this destiny, through the self-determination of Karma Yoga, is possible through the knowledge obtained in the making of a Shiva Lingam. Understanding the components of form and energy, understanding the interconnectedness of all things, understanding our vulnerability to force, and our ability to exert force, gives power to utilize this knowledge and obtain whatever is desired. Do not pray for what is needed or wanted - understanding the causes that give rise to the conditions of success (or failure), confidently act to condition success and decondition failure: do not pray for protection, or refuge, but act promptly to bring an end to what is threatening you.

The name of Parvati connotes a rock, or stone - as the daughter of the mountains or even the Shiva Lingam; it connotes what is beyond (para-), what fulfills and fills and is suitable (parv-), what was asked for or begged (vati-). Thus, since you know better than to pray, since you know that all Lingas will eventually be destroyed, like an icicle in the spring, the Linga is by extended practice made to appear formless: grasp sand with two hands and clasp it between those hands. Let it go: and it falls to the ground, formless, even dispersed on the wind. This is the Shiva Lingam. Grasp mud with two hands and clasp it between those hands. Let it go: it forms a small formless pillar that through time is observed to disperse. This is the Shiva Lingam. So is a rock, unshaped except by the gradual processes of water, wind, ice, and other natural phenomenon, grasped in the hands: this is also the Shiva Lingam. Curl in despair, and cower, holding your legs and back with your hands, in a fetal position weep and cry like Shiva in His grief at the death of Sati: this, your body, is also the Shiva Lingam. Your sorrow will eventually pass, and you will stand up straight, like a pillar. This is also the Shiva Lingam.

The three gunas are present in all things, present in the Shiva Linga. Grasping this, as you would grasp one of your hands with the other to make a Shiva Lingam, as you grasp the subtle nature of reality - and your own nature as well - say "Om Namah Shivaya!" It is by Yoga that Shiva is realized.

Excerpts from the Shiva Lingam Purana

After sense, after perception of sense, after consciousness of perception, after awareness of consciousness, after understanding of awareness, after all knowledge that comes from such information is what lies before that knowing - what is before is also after. As an egg is non-separate from the bird, insect or other being that emerges from within it, the egg resulting in the birth of another egg - as a being results in further beings, so does sensation and information result in more information and sensation; so does knowledge result in more knowledge. A circle has no beginning or ending, except the point at which it is first discovered or described. All information shapes the way it is interpreted into knowledge. A pillar, if it might be extended indefinitely, would circle back upon itself, as you would hold yourself in your own arms tightly to touch hand to hand - so does all becoming encircle its own conditions of beginning and ending: this encircling, this holding onto of information and sense, this discovery and description, this declaration, this pillar - this is the emergence of Shiva. Shiva emerges from this thing, this pillar, this line or causation, this reasoning upon information, this linga. This is the symbol of Shiva.

The linga is made to appear formless: grasp sand with two hands and clasp it between those hands. Let it go: and it falls to the ground, formless, even dispersed on the wind. This is the Shiva Lingam. Grasp mud with two hands and clasp it between those hands. Let it go: it forms a small formless pillar that through time is observed to disperse. This is the Shiva Lingam. So is a rock, unshaped except by the gradual processes of water, wind, ice, and other natural phenomenon, grasped in the hands: this is also the Shiva Lingam. The three gunas are present in all things, present in the Shiva Linga. Grasping this, as you would grasp one of your hands with the other to make a Shiva Lingam, say "Om Namah Shivaya!" It is by Yoga that Shiva is realized.

Color (especially red), white and black are used to symbolically express Raja, Sattva, and Tamas respectively. These are present in all things, to greater or lesser degree - not because they elementally form all things, but are the emergent property of things. As Vishnu is an emergent property of discovering what has been declared by Brahma, as Brahma is an emergent property of declaring what has been discovered, so are both emergent properties of Shiva - and Shiva emerges from discovery and declaration. There cannot be made distinction which comes first, or second: the infinite pillar forms a circle and has no top or bottom, no beginning or ending, no first or second. No distinction in honor or priority can be made between parent and child, between fetus and womb, between hatchling, mother and egg.

Once, Brahma and Vishnu came to violent disagreement which had come first: but then a flaming pillar separated them. This pillar of Shiva, the Shiva Lingam, challenged the both of them to find its beginning or end, to exceed it. So Brahma and Vishnu each sought their own domain. Brahma flew upward into space like a swan, and Vishnu directed himself downward through space, as a boar digs into the earth: Vishnu sought to discover the foundation of the pillar, Brahma sought to find the extent of the pillar. And both exhausted themselves before finding the limits of the pillar: for it circled back onto itself without end or beginning. Blinded by the flames, neither Brahma nor Vishnu were aware that the other similarly struggled, or even of their own endless circling: to them, the pillar remained straight, and infinite - while Vishnu flew one direction on the interior of the circle and Brahma on the exterior in the opposite direction they crossed paths, but didn't even know it. When both Brahma and Vishnu each understood they had failed, when they had stilled, and quieted, they heard the pillar: "a-u-m" Om! They saw on the pillar the letters a-u-m. They saw the pillar formed those letters. A-U-M are, respectively, the sounds/letters of Brahma, Vishnu and Shiva. They knew the pillar to be Shiva, and their mistake in seeking primacy. Shiva said, "we are all three part of the same, the act of beginning conditions the act of preservation and sustaining - as well as ending. The act of preservation and sustaining condition its ending, and its beginning. The act of ending conditions beginning and sustaining. Do not fight yourself, you will only exhaust yourself."

One grows filthy from exertion and work to require a bath, and bathes for work. One rests to prepare for work that will require additional rest. It is by making vows we learn not to, it is by taking up that we let go. One learns from a teacher to exceed that teacher, and become teacherless. By understanding the limits of sense and knowledge, one comprehends logic, and reality.

The altar of the Shiva Lingam (Shakti Yoni) is representative of Uma. The exterior of the Shiva Lingam is representative of Brahma, the center of the lingam is representative of Vishnu. One should only undertake the practices of Shiva Lingam with no teacher.

Raja Yoga: a duty of preparation

Besides clearing the room of stones, fire, water, filth and otherwise preparing it for practice, Swami Swatmarama said Hatha can only be perfected "in a country where justice is properly administered, where good people live, and food can be obtained easily and plentifully." This basic preparation for Hatha Yoga is the simplest expression of the essence of Raja Yoga.

The Yogi must prepare the room - and the country in which it is situated - for their practice.

Fire preparation

The Buddha described the preparation made for fire, saying,

Suppose you want to make a small fire into a large fire: if you put wet fuel on it, expose it to wind and rain, or sprinkle it with dust, will that make the small fire grow? Just so, the mind requires proper fuel and conditions for enlightenment: tranquility, peace and equanimity. These three conditions can wake a sluggish mind. How are these conditions achieved? Through curiosity, will and energetic exertion, and playful love or friendship.

And what are the conditions for tranquility, curiosity, will and energetic exertion, and playful love or friendship? These are the conditions of enlightenment (bojjihanga - limbs of enlightenment, so-called because they lead to enlightenment): mindfulness (sati-sambojjangha), understanding of mental and physical natures (dhamma-vicaya-s, connoting "science"), exertion or energy (viriya-s), playful love or friendship (piiti-s, different than Sukha - happiness, contentment), tranquility (passaddhi-s), peace (samaadhi-s), equanimity (upekkhaa-s).

Suppose you want to start a fire: if you have only wet fuel, if it is windy and rainy, if you sprinkle it with dust, will you be able to start a fire?

Those are the wrong conditions to start a fire. Just so, when a mind is agitated it is the wrong time to wake it to enlightenment. A new fire is easily extinguished, but a large fire is not. It is difficult to wake, it is more difficult to wake to enlightenment, but it is even more difficult to extinguish the flame of enlightenment.

And what is the condition for extinguishing agitation, to permit sluggishness to be roused into wakefulness? Mindfulness. Mindfulness is always useful, in every circumstance, whereas the other conditions are only sometimes appropriate.

The limits of ethics and necessity in ritual: Bhakti Yoga

As a person might draw on a 2-dimensional paper an image of a sphere, but may never truthfully say "this is a sphere," nor would be incorrect in saying "this is a sphere," nor could this person in reality form a perfect sphere even in 3-dimensions to truly call it "a sphere," or even draw a perfect circle in 2 dimensions to truly call it "a circle," the Puranas are illustrative of theoretical concepts which cannot be otherwise demonstrated. Understanding this is the ultimate purpose of the Puranas: understanding that truth is itself a theoretical abstraction is essential to understanding the conditional relevance and necessity of falsehoods: sometimes a lie is necessary, or irrelevant.

A wheel sometimes need not be entirely perfectly round to provide a smooth ride: some roads are rougher, and it won't matter whether the wheel is well balanced. The measure of good conscience may be made only after discovering the extent to which the demands of morality are flexible.

What, then, is the fixed measure of conscience?

Sometimes an athlete needs a competitor - but not all games are measured by the achievements of a challenger: for in a weak challenger, the bar is held too low. Thus, some games are won by your own strength or speed, alone. It is when we are alone that we find our truest challenge, and understand there is no need for an antagonist or protagonist. This is true in game and sport, as well as in industry and art, and especially in matters of political administration.

Frequently, a person may even believe in a god - fervently - that another does not believe in. To an observer who either believes in still a different god, or no god at all, both beliefs seem foolish. Yet even such an absurd premise should not be engaged, but accepted and respected. The politics, economics, philosophy, flags, heroes, and other sacred things and ways of doing things of an opponent should be venerated as if they were our own: these precious things represent the culmination of numerous facts and experience, they are symbols of the principles which are mutually shared and therefore are irrelevant to the present disagreement. And, it is bad form, not to mention counterproductive and improper, to argue over that which has already been agreed upon.

Games may be won or lost by knowing and following the rules. But life is not a game: it has no rules to know, and freed from the construct of morality, it is clear one may do everything "right" and still lose. It is simply irrelevant to consider the motivations of an action: right or wrong, moral or immoral, the effects are the same. Frequently, the best intentions result badly.

Therefore, in fighting, it is possible to mistake a friend for an opponent when ideologically opposed: even ideological opposites share common interests, and benefit from mutual assistance toward these goals. Indeed, even within a one camp or another, facts and experience are gathered, agendas shift, ideologies shift, and political affiliations shift - no doubt about it, such a world of change can be a source of anxiety. All beings seek safety from this changing world. And seeking safety, we would attack what seems to give us fear, and put down challengers to our own puissance, thinking "reduce the measure of our contest, and we more easily succeed. If our competitor does worse, the easier we shall do better!"

But this strategy fails because there is a fixed measure of success. No attack on a challenger can change the true measure of success, we are not competing against one another, no matter our belief otherwise.

Fighting with our friends and neighbors will not make us better, nor more secure. Ignoring our friends and neighbors so they feel like they have to yell to be heard (and still not being heard when they yell) is not securing ourselves against doubt. It is possible in such strategy to become so acutely aware of our opponents' faults as to become blinded to our own. And holding absent-mindedly and inflexibly to our own wrong beliefs, act against our own interests.

Consider instead that the measure of good conscience is known only by discovering the limitations of morality. And especially reflect on how those who have measured the limits of morality frequently find them wanting. What seems cautious to one will undoubtedly seem callous and cowardly to another. But is is not our duty to be cautious, or bold. It is our duty to love, and in such athletics of the heart as our nature guides us, to succeed. Success comes not through difficulty or ease alone, but by remembering what is easy, what is our nature, our dharma, we may strive to improve. Flexing our only a little, we will not find our reach lacks strength. Remembering what is our duty, we will not hesitate to act: remembering what is the duty of others we will be better content to permit them to also strive. They do not challenge us, nor threaten us. There is no cause for jealousy: those who fail to reach the summit of their ambition frequently find honor enough in lending a hand to those who press behind. The drum inspires heroes, even when beaten to pieces. It is not in winning, but in the athletic effort itself, that we find satisfaction of our purpose.

Sacrifice the score and you will enjoy the game better. Sacrifice your win: friendship with the other players is better prized. In such boisterous enthusiasm, you will exert yourself and discover your limits - are boundless. Sacrifice, and love, Kama - by these strategies there is success. Play for honor, and you will certainly succeed.

Practice Bhakti if you would have your sacrifice be meaningful.

Forehead ornamentation

The practice of forehead ornamentation originated out of the practice of making shiva lingams as described in the Lingam Purana: making one's hands, head and/or other parts of or the entire body a lingam was ritually signified by decorating it as such. This practice was quickly adopted by Vaishnavas, and other devotees, becoming a ceremony of Bhakti Yoga: these non-Shaivites were not making "lingams," but used other symbology and rituals common to their own practices.

But all these marks, once intended to be a symbol of impermanence, have left emotional and cultural scars. And it is in seeing these scars, and a rejection of all symbolic marks, that the achievement of their original purpose may be found.

As the practices were developed and explored, the symbols necessarily took on additional meanings. During the several occupations of India, these symbols were utilized first as a way of distinguishing between various practitioners of Yoga, and then encouraged as a method by which Yogis might differentiate themselves from each other: sects were formed and politicized, dividing the people so that they might be easier to dominate. Thus, these symbols became gradually associated with the Brahman varna (and the varnas themselves became a caste into which one was born, rather than attained with training, association and practice) at the same time that Yoga was encouraged to become more a centralized and organized religion (also to aid the occupations): what originally was intended as a marking of a Yogi undertaking Priestly duties necessarily changed when "Priest" became an occupation to which a Yogi would devote themselves to entirely, and practice, and even inherit. Thus, ironically, the use of ash, or other powders intended to be very impermanent and liberating, easily manufactured to encourage the access of any person, were twisted into the support of a permanent and oppressive caste system, and to the exclusion of the majority of Yogis for the purpose of supporting a centralized and organized method of control. The timeframe of this transformation was very long: things changed slowly, and subtly. It has been a long time since the occupation ended: these tikas have persisted, and continue to take new symbolic meaning, both because of and in response to the emergent Hindu nationalist movement that brought about an end to the occupation.

The originally simplistic symbols were given complexity by rounding or curving lines and edges, or ornamenting the terminal points of lines: coloration and spacing became very important, as well. Each variant became associated with different practices and expressed different association. And sometimes are combined, to symbolize mutual association and recognition. A u-shaped arc became associated with the Swamis who flourished during the British occupation during the late 18th Century: these Swamis professed a practice that was conducive to centralization, organization, and allegiance that the governors encouraged. The long history of the monastic movement (dating back to the 6th century), and its rejection of Buddhism, and other pan-Hinduism, is too long to be simply remarked on here: it suffices to express that they developed their own symbology, and their use of this symbology encouraged others to adopt different and similar symbology.

Shaivites continue to utilize a basic form of three horizontal lines (as on a lingam). Vaishnavas continue to utilize a basic form of vertical lines. Swamis continue to use the U-shaped arc. Shaktas continue to utilize a dot. And so forth: circles, triangles, squares, arcs, crescents, crosses, and so many variants! Honorary association typically is typically signified by a simplistic rendition of these basic forms. And there is also an expression of no-mark, a blank forehead, a rejection of the entire practice wherein decorations are only rarely used, or not used at all.

As these forms were abstracted and complicated, there also arose a counter-movement toward the use of these decorations by non-Brahmans, both as a socio-political expression against the occupation's caste system and central organization, and also as a way of expressing casual association or alliance with the various groups using these symbols.

The Bindi, or purely decorative mark, whether in the form of a jewel or precious powder (makeup), arose as a stylistic expression of this counter-reaction. The no-mark also arose from this counter-reaction: the restoration of practices by which it is through self-control and effort that one becomes a Brahman, capable of Priestly duties of sacrifice, the rejection that only Brahmans are capable of sacrifice and other Priestly duties, seemed to require rejecting what became a symbol contrary to these practices and celebrating what is uniquely symbolic of other Varna - it was a way of expressing a rejection of all Varna, an expression of the sacrifice of Varna. Additionally, as the Swamic rejection of Buddhism was itself rejected, Buddhist practices of no-marking were adopted - for various reasons. Even as some Buddhists adopted the practice of marking their foreheads with symbols of their own.

Today, the reason a person bears these marks is highly personal - sometimes to express one thing or another, or nothing at all. The highly radical practices of jewelled bindis has become (to a great degree) entirely secular practice, as unsymbolic as merely decorating the face with lipstick or dying the hair. Or as a cultural statement.

How do you decorate yourself? When? And why?

The best puja

In the performance of puja, we cannot blame a person for making a deity or religion their favorite as long as the person acknowledges that all theology and atheology is in fact the same - not any more than we might blame a person for preferring one flavor of food over another, or a particular kind of clothing to another, or a form of housing to another, or even one land to another. Preference itself is no fault, for there is greater or lesser suitability to our ability and purpose in the infinite diversity of our choices. However, to be fooled by the illusion of differences we have imagined when presented with choices of essential similarity, to ignore the irrelevancy of such subtlety by turning from the pragmatism of our logic, or to forget our own individuality by thinking that what is suitable to ourselves is suitable to another, is a profound fault. Each individual is sacred, for it is an indivisible part of the whole. What difference is there between one and all? Between none and one? Between yours and mine? Between you and me? Such differences are of our own making - and yet, if we are controlled by them, it is arguably no longer a useful tool, but an implement of our own harm.

What beliefs we cannot sacrifice are not ours, but control us - and it is our obligation to free ourselves from them.

In the long war between the Devas and Asuras, each would occasionally conquer the world of the other, and then retake their home; appealing for help sometimes to Vishnu, sometimes to Shiva, sometimes to Brahma, sometimes to Shakti - and other non-beings - the opponents were restored to balance for a time as these non-beings took one form or another required for a temporary victory. Yet because of the fundamental nature of each opponent was so contrary to the other that they inevitably found themselves in conflict again: when they were victorious, they would forget their prior defeats and the help they had received; when they were defeated, they would forget their prior victories, and grow angry in their sulking.

When, once more, Vishnu was asked for help from the Devas after the Asuras had taken the Devaloka from them, and asked by the Asuras for help because the Devas had taken the Asuraloka from them, He understood the problem lay in this fundamental nature of things. What was required was for the asuras to willingly release what they took - but past experience suggested they would be utterly unwilling to do this. Yet, understanding the more fundamental nature of each individual being (even the Asuras) was toward an evolution of existence by several Ashrams, Vishnu instead devoted His effort to the growth and strengthening of the Asuras. Yet Vishnu found he was not Himself developed sufficiently, and devoted Himself toward personal growth.

The Devas were, reasonably, confused how any of this was helping their cause. Yet when, at last, Vishnu attained enlightenment, and began to teach Sannyasa, they saw the Asuras lay down all that they had taken up - even the Vedas themselves. Such a Vedasamnyasa was not atheism, and

Vishnu could not teach contrary to the Vedas, being a manifestation of them. Such non-theism was the natural result of spiritual practice.

When the Devas retook their Devaloka, and the Asuras too returned home, it was not by conquest; there was nothing to inflame their pride and reignite the war. The Devas and the Asuras had taken up the Buddhist practices of Vishnu and outgrown their struggle; turning inward, they faced their true enemy, and changed their nature. Changing their own nature, they changed the nature of the world, and a new age began. In a sign of His growth, even King Indra personally attended to the Buddha, humbly, as any simple monk might, peacefully, side by side, with His former enemies. They had all given up everything - even their enmity.

Can you, too, give up your fighting, and relinquish both heaven and hell

Stories for Bhakti: Shiva

Nandi - the vehicle

Nandi is the vehicle of Shiva, and also the vehicle of Gauri. As well as the vehicle of the Matrikas, the nurse mothers of Shiva and Parvati's son Kartikeya.

But more, Nandi is Shiva.

It is probably best to start with what a "vehicle" is: a "vehicle" (or Vahana) is that which "carries" or "transports." In this sense, a vehicle is the means by which the being or existence of Shiva manifests. A "being" is devoid of "force," "power" or "identity." It is the "presence" which the vehicle carries: much as a truck, or a horse, acting as a vehicle, might carry or transport your presence. A vehicle is how you navigate space - and this is exactly what Shiva uses Nandi for.

Shiva, like Vishnu, or Brahma, etc., are not adequately described in terms of space, or time. Or existence. But when existent, Shiva bears force, power, identity, and occupies and traverses space and time. While other vehicles are distinct from that which they are carrying and transporting (Ganesh's vehicle is a mouse, for example), it is not so unusual to use yourself as a vehicle: many people, and most animals, walk there or here on their own feet.

Shiva does not have feet, per-se. But Shiva does have Nandi.

In the Linga Purana 17.3.4, Shilad greatly pleased Shiva by his devotion (which lasted for thousands of years). Shiva wanted to reciprocate the devotion to his devotee, and asked Shilad what he most desired? Shilad said, a self-born and immortal son. Shiva knew what Shilad was getting at: Shilad's devotion to Shiva was like that of a parent for a child - a practice very much like Vatsalya Bhava. Shiva acknowledged Brahma had been trying to convince Shiva to take form again. "I will take birth as your son, and my name will be Nandi. And I shall give you immortality."

In the Kurma Purana 12.33, Shilada was plowing, an act of Yajna Kunda, the land when suddenly a handsome boy appeared on top of the plow! The boy could speak, and called Shilada "Father." The boy, Nandi, studied the shastras and became very learned. Nandi wished nothing more than to see Shiva. And to become immortal, like his father - whom he loved very much. Sitting on the shores of the ocean, he called out to Shiva thousands of times. At last, Shiva appeared (remember that Shiva exists beyond space and time, and so appearing to a form Shiva took is not necessarily more complicated than when a person talks to themselves out loud). Nandi was delighted! Shiva asked Nandi what Nandi wanted? Nandi said, "grant me enough life to call your name out thousands of times more, and see you again!" This was granted. And again and again, Nandi devoted himself to Shiva. But Shiva knew what Nandi actually wanted. The third time, Shiva appeared with Parvati and said "Enough is enough - there is no need to keep calling out My name to see Me. I will make you the guardian of my gates, you shall be my vehicle, you shall be Lord of all the Ganas. You shall be my constant companion!" Shiva then arranged a marriage between Nandi and Suyasha.

But why was Nandi so concerned with death? The Shatrudra Samhita 5.3 describes the Yajna Kunda in which Nandi appeared resulted in tremendous celebration. Shiva and Parvati both arrived to bless the child (again, as both Shiva and Parvati do not exist within time or space, this is no great obstacle to understanding). Visitors kept coming, though - to celebrate. Even seven years later! (People traveled slowly back then). At last, one day, to Brahmans came and informed Shilad that after one year, Nandi would cease to be. Shilad understood this to be "dead" and grew very upset, very sad. After all - he loved his son, and Shiva had promised an immortal child? Seeing his father so upset, Nandi quickly learned what was said. Nandi wished nothing more than to see Shiva - but now also wanted to become immortal, and fulfill his father's faith and desire. When Shiva had told Nandi he would be Shiva's constant companion, and never die, Shiva said "you are just like me, so you will never die." Just because something or someone ceases to be does not mean they die!

Shiva gave to Nandi one of his garlands, and as soon as Nandi put on that garland, Nandi imbibed all the qualities of Shiva. Which is fortunate, because at the "beginning" of things when the poison of Karma spilt across the universe, Nandi was there, beyond space and time, by Shiva's side to drink the poison that dribbled from Shiva's mouth. Like Shiva, Nandi was not killed by the poison, either. And Nandi was guarding Shiva's gates when Gauri asked him to keep everyone out while Gauri bathed - and because Nandi permitted Shiva to enter despite Gauri's order (Nandi could not refuse Shiva anything, since Nandi WAS Shiva), Gauri eventually made Ganesh. Ganesh is known as a Lord of the Ganas, too. But Nandi is the first Gana, and out of penance for disobeying Gauri in preference for Shiva, gives fresh grass to Ganesh annually as a gift (grass is something both Nandi - who is a "bull" - and Ganesh - who is an "elephant" - enjoy). In other stories, Nandi teaches great Gurus - and has many adventures of his own.

You can usually see a picture or statue of Nandi guarding the gates of Shiva's shrines. These usually are seated, facing the main shrine. Nandi is a master of joy, happiness, and kama. He is a master of music and dance.

It is interesting to realize, however, that Shiva is both consort and vehicle to his "wife." This indicates in a special way the unique relationship that develops through love. And that special relationship, that special love, is extended to the nurse mothers of his child, too.

Hanuman - the Bhakti

Hanuman is also known as the "son of the Wind," but the wind merely carried Shiva's ejaculate to the womb of his wife, Anjana. To mature the seed, both took the form of Vanaras. Thus, Hanuman was borne to the form of a Vanara as well.

The Vanara (literally a term that means both "is it a human?" [vav-nara] and "forest people" [vana-nara]) are often portrayed as proto-human monkeys: due to the extreme age of the story, these stories may in fact contain the impressions our ancestors had of the several species (now-extinct) of other hominids that co-inhabited lands together.

The stories are filled with numerous similar forms of parentage: when a person desired children, and could not otherwise obtain pregnancy, they availed themselves of surrogacy (if the female was infertile or subfertile), insemination (if the male was infertile or subfertile), or adoption (adoption was undertaken for other reasons, as well: compassion, not least among them). The relationship of parent and child, like that of spouses and even consorts, was one which was entered into by choice, or a purpose.

Beyond time and space, Shiva's "brother" Vishnu had taken female form of Mohini to attack the Asuras in defense of the Devas. Mohini's weapon was seduction (the only weapon to which the Asuras were vulnerable at that moment), but Vishnu was uncertain of whether s/he had mastered the weapon, as Vishnu had not yet used it. So, Mohini asked Shiva to permit a challenge: Shiva's self-control was beyond comparison, and if Mohini could seduce Shiva, then Mohini had nothing to worry about in her attack on the Asuras. Shiva instantly was seduced, and called for the help of Gauri, Shiva's ardhangini. Even with Gauri's help, Shiva could not withstand Mohini. Gauri even merged with Shiva, and even in this bisexual/asexual state, Shiva could not withstand Mohini. Thus, Hanuman may be understood to be the product of Mohini's victory. That Mohini could not become pregnant at that time (Vishnu was going off to war, after all) did not mean that the seed should be wasted: Vayu rescued the semen before it fell to the earth, and both Vayu and Anjana being a devotee of Shiva, and Vishnu, they desired to mature that seed.

The name "Hanuman" connotes the destruction of pride: Shiva was utterly defeated and humiliated by Vishnu. Hanuman's humility is one of his greatest assets in all his challenges: understanding he is limited in his ability to grow stronger and smarter, understanding his limitations, he is able to work around them. He is famous for generalizations (like bringing a mountain of herbs when he did not know how to identify the correct one needed), and non-methodical leaps across oceans and voids - and logic. His undefeated persistence earns him success. He is loyal, and loving, being unable, it is by humbly serving those who are able that he earns greater honor than he might on his own - and gains greater ability than they have.

By the end of his life he has mastered every art and science - simply because he was willing to learn them. And throughout his life, he is drawn toward and loves Vishnu (Rama).

Shiva Purana 11 - the friend

Vishnu gave to Shiva a garland of santanaka flowers to give as a gift to Indra, King of the Devas, who had just won a war between the Asuras and Devas. Indra had thought he had finally conquered every world from the Asuras, and did not yet understand that this meant his war would continue: he could not yet comprehend the means to peace with the Asuras - or that Vishnu could be a friend to both the Asuras and the Devas. The flowers were given as a gift to "celebrate" his victory, and help the Asuras. Indra graciously accepted the flowers, and draped them around the neck of his vehicle, the elephant Airavata. But there were bees on the flower, and the animal grew terrified: Airavata pulled off the flowers and smashed them (and the bees) on the ground.

Shiva played the part Vishnu cast him, and spoke in anger (though of course this reaction of Airavata is exactly what was intended from the start), "arrogant Indra! Even if it were just a gift from me, you shouldn't treat it like this! That was a gift from Vishnu! Now look what you have done to it! You will lose the three worlds you rule, you will lose all your wealth. And all your devas will experience old age and death!" Airavata, being Indra's vehicle, was more than a simple elephant: it was an extension of Indra's own person, and Shiva had every right to be upset. Indra tried to apologize, but Shiva coldly said "I am not forgiving!" echoing Indra's own words when the Asuras had begged forgiveness.

Proud Indra, though he understood, did not make things right. So, when the next war between the Asuras and Devas came, the Devas actually died from the Asura's weapons. To Indra's surprise, the Devas did not come back to life as they usually had! And all the Devas began to weaken from their extreme age. The Devas quickly lost every world to the Asuras. They sought the help of Brahma, who was aware of Vishnu's play. Brahma therefore advised them to seek the help of Vishnu. Vishnu was their friend, after all.

Vishnu said he would help the Devas, he was their friend, after all. "Devas, churn the Kshirasagara (primordial ocean), until it gives up amrita (a word that means "no longer begging for what sustains life" a thing which satisfies every desire - - it is a play on words, as well, as the Devas had been reduced to beggars, and were begging Vishnu for forgiveness). Let the Asuras be your allies in the churning - at least until the amrita rises. Agree to any condition they demand, and I promise you none of them will drink the amrita. Befriend them - as the snake does the mouse."

(The reason for not sharing the amrita lies in both previous and subsequent episodes of this story, of which this section is only one episode - but suffice to say that the Asuras already had Amrita, though they did not know it. Eventually, Vishnu, by the last several Avataras, restores peace to both Asuras and Devas: it is not by conquest or domination one establishes peace, but by accomplishing the purpose of the struggle, and working with an adversary against the conditions that led to opposition. Vishnu teaches both sides self-restraint, and to sacrifice both their right to revenge and victory, teaching them to value the friendship and cooperation they sought enough to remember it was their purpose. Thus, the Devas and Asuras sacrifice not only the worlds they conquered, but their native worlds too - for the sake of the friendship and peace they rightly desired because they understood the means of conflict and war was not accomplishing their purpose: this is how they all became friends, living in peace, together with all the beings of every world. Vishnu, eventually, by the subsequent Avatara of the Buddha, shares the Amrita with all beings).

So Indra led the Devas to Bali, the Asura King. They lied, just as Vishnu had directed them to and Bali was convinced that his victory over them and every world would not be complete without the amrita - and those other things which would emerge from the churning. "Neither the Asuras nor Devas alone have the strength to churn the ocean, but together we might." As they began to plan how to do this great thing, Vishnu spoke to the assembly of Devas and Asuras, saying "use Mount Madara as your churning rod, and Vasuki and his people as your rope." (Vasuki was the King of the Nagas, dragon or snake-like beings who could change shape at will, and a servant-vehicle of Vishnu).

Of course, Vasuki was in on the play as well, and agreed to be used as a rope when Bali offered him a share of the Amrita, and commanded all his people to be used as ropes as well. So the Devas and Asuras, singing in their work, uprooted Mount Madara and tried to carry it to the ocean - but it was too heavy, and they dropped it, killing many Devas and Asuras. The survivors began to cry, and so Vishnu cheered them up - with one finger, he lifted Mandara, and revived all the dead Asuras and Devas. As if helping children with their work, Vishnu completed the task of bringing the mountain to the ocean.

Vasuki and his people wound themselves around the mountain, and announced they were ready. The Devas took hold of the head, and the Asuras the tail - and the Asuras protested - they would not be denied the honor of the greater danger (Vasuki breathed fire, and in the exertion could not be expected to fully restrain himself). Vishnu smiled, sighed, shook his head at this arrogance and encouraged the Devas, "agree to whatever the Asuras want." So the Devas and Asuras switched places.

The mountain kept sinking down into the ocean's floor, and so they could not churn the ocean. So, Vishnu was manifested by Kurma, the turtle, and swimming to the ocean floor, supported the churning rod. Now, the Asuras and Devas sang and enjoyed the work, greater and greater speed, stirring the sea like you would make cheese out of milk. Vishnu laughed and enjoyed the friendship the Asuras and Devas shared, and because he was tickled by the spinning mountain on his back.

But the faster the churning, the more the mountain wobbled. So Vishnu was manifested again, thousand armed as tall as the sky, and held the peak of the mountain steady. Now, Vishnu was above and below the mountain, as well as the churning rope. But the Asuras and Devas were playing together, in friendship: they challenged one another to greater exertion, and effort, in love.

But now the trouble started: Vasuki was strained, and began to vomit fire and venom, this burned Bali, and the other Asuras. All their fancy clothes and garlands were burned, their jewelry was scalded by the acid. Of course, the Devas were more resistant to it, and this suffering was unnecessary. Nevertheless, the Asuras refused to yield their position to the Devas. By their stubbornness, the Asuras would have been burned alive, but Vishnu then manifested as a thundershower, and cooled the flames. The waters began to froth, and things began to rise out of the waves.

Now the Asuras and Devas were growing tired. So Vishnu manifested on either end of their long line holding Vasuki, as both a Deva and Asura, and as a parent would secretly aid their children in a difficult task, secretly lent his strength to the churning. Vishnu was able to keep his help secret because when the Devas and Asuras grew tired, they were also helped by every other being - this helped the Devas and Asuras confuse the strength of Vishnu with their own.

(It should be clear by now that Vishnu might have churned the ocean by himself. But only the Devas and Asuras could build their own friendship).

Now the fish fled the area: the halahala (poison) began to rise from the ancient ocean floor, threatening to hurt Vishnu - and destroy every world by ending Time (Vishnu is Time). Vishnu began to worry: only Shiva could save him from the halahala: Vishnu called out to Shiva to take the poison, "Shiva accepts everything!" Sacrificing the poison to Shiva, Vishnu sacrificed his own defeat: in the nick of time, Shiva commanded the Ganas to gather the poison, and Shiva drank it all up. Gauri, his literal "other half" manifested as Bhavani, and choked him, so that the poison would not enter his body, or leave his mouth, but stay in his throat until it could be purified. Nandi, his vehicle and extension, licked up the drops of poison that dribbled from Shiva's mouth before they caused much harm.

Now the ocean began to yield its treasures: Kamadhenu (a wish-granting cow), Varuni (intoxication), Ucchaisravas (a horse-vehicle of light, the Apsaras, the moon, and much more. Both the Devas and Asuras equally received great treasure from the churning, and even gave each other gifts of the treasures they were earning in expressions of friendship and love. This delighted Vishnu.

But then, just as Vishnu was growing too tired to continue his work (remember, the Asuras and Devas were "helping" Vishnu, but not enough to actually accomplish the churning), he manifested Dhanvantari, a manifestation of medicine as a physician, bearing Amrita, and Vishnu thus tended his own strain and wounds. And that of the Devas and Asuras too. The churning continued.

Now, they exerted a little more and from their "second wind" of determination out of the ocean rose Laxmi, Vishnu's love and wife. In this moment of her re-making, she did not recognize where she was for a moment, or anything about her: then she saw Vishnu, and remembering her love for him, went to his side, as if she had always been there. She then helped in the churning, sitting atop the mountain (which is now on every side of Vishnu), she brought the Ganga, and all the rivers, and precious fruits, and dance, and all kinds of other refreshment, rest and recreation, to renew everyone's effort. The Vedas were chanted, and the work continued - but then the Asuras saw that Dhanvantari, the physician, was using the amrita to treat everyone!

(See how Vishnu had tricked the Asuras and Devas to keep working, after the amrita rose - so that Laxmi might be churned out of the ocean?).

The Asuras began to fight over the amrita, and could not decide who should drink first, or how much share everyone should get. But then suddenly, they became aware of an embodiment of Seduction: Vishnu manifested as Mohini, and approached. Bali was overcome by Seduction and mindlessly gave the amrita to Mohini, "please, share this among us as would be fair?"

Mohini studied the Asuras carefully, as if about to attack them. Then she said, "I am Seduction. Haven't you heard that I am dangerous? And yet you think I am your friend? You come near to me, and stay by me, and even ask my help? So be it. I will help you - but only if you do whatever I say, whether or not it seems right or wrong." The Asuras, totally overcome by Seduction, agreed.

Mohini made the Devas and Asuras assemble in a hall, which was made to be as romantic as possible. There, she continued her work of seduction, and the Asuras and Devas grew insane with desire. Mohini's loose clothes occasionally slipped, revealing everything; she flirted with the Asuras, and promised them everything. Then, when the Asuras were sufficiently crazed, she was satisfied: they were utterly defeated by her seduction, when they understood this, they would be humiliated. So she sat the Asuras on one side, and the Devas on the other. She poured the Amrita for the Devas first, taking her time, while looking over her shoulder at the Asuras, and flirting with the Asuras. Though the Asuras were now quite impatient, they waited, not wanting to upset Mohini. Except Rahu.

Rahu, the Asura, saw the trick of Mohini, and made himself appear like a Deva. He snuck across the hall to sit with the Devas, between the Surya (sun) and Soma (moon). Mohini was too distracted by her work of seduction to notice that Rahu was not what he seemed - until Surya and Soma cried out! In an instant, Rahu drank the Amrita, and in the same instant, Mohini drew a Chakra (a frisbee-like razor weapon, which is associated with Vishnu) and cut off Rahu's head - but because he had already tasted the Amrita, Rahu's head was immortal. Rahu flew off into the sky, and Vishnu recognized Rahu's achievement, and permitted him that victory. Yet even today, Rahu, Soma and Surya continue their squabble, and occasionally, Rahu will eclipse them, though frequently Soma and Surya chase Rahu from the sky.

The Asuras did not even notice this chaotic event, so taken were they with Mohini. It was not until the Devas had drunk all the Amrita that the Asuras noticed none was left for them. Vishnu took his usual form. Realizing they had been tricked, the Asuras attacked the Devas - and Vishnu. Vishnu, with a firm gentleness and kindness, drove them back until the domains of the Devas and Asuras were restored to how they were before the wars. But, in chasing the Asuras to their home, Mohini herself was lost to the insanity of seduction: the Asuras were quick learners, and had learned Seduction from Vishnu! In Patala, their home, the Asuras and their wives and husbands now seduced Vishnu, capturing Vishnu!

Vishnu, still as Mohini, had practiced seduction, but unwisely, not practiced the defense against seduction. In response, she used the only weapon in her hand: and counter attacking seduction with seduction, the Asuras and Vishnu were driven insane. Thus, Vishnu would have remained in Patala forever, ensnared by desire, if Shiva had not followed after Vishnu and tried to rescue him. Both Mohini and her captors attacked Shiva - in the insanity, no one wanted Vishnu to leave! The Devas chased after Shiva to try to rescue Shiva, but then themselves became overcome by desire in the seduction of Mohini and all the Asuras. After the Devas came the Yakshas, Rakshasas, and all the other beings of every world - each would-be rescuer themselves overcome. Soon, every being was then in Patala, writhing in desire. Even Shiva began to weaken. Shiva understood what needed to be done - but before he himself was overcome, he had to destroy Mohini's beautiful form.

At last, for a moment, the trance was broken, and Shiva was able to carry Vishnu, and all the beings of every world, back to where they all belonged. Vishnu apologized, and Shiva forgave him - Vishnu was not invincible, after all. Shiva warned everyone to stay away from Patala - it was not a place easy to escape from!

Mohini, of course, had other adventures before this, and many other adventures afterward: Vishnu is Time, and not bound by Time. Previously, Shiva helped Vishnu perfect the form of Mohini, permitting Vishnu to test the weapons of seduction on him before using them on the Asuras and Devas (Vishnu thought that if Shiva could be overpowered, he, Vishnu, could overpower anyone). And even with the help of Gauri, Shiva could not withstand Mohini - and when Shiva spontaneously lost control of his semen, it was taken by the wind to his wife, and Hanuman was born. When Gauri could not restrain Shiva, Shiva captured Mohini, and they coupled: from this coupling, Ayappan the tiger-rider was born.

But those other stories cannot be told here, without confusing digression.

So, now, the Devas believed they had again triumphed, and this was the end to war. Shiva saw this, and approached them, and tried to help them: he showed them how, from the beginning, Vishnu had set them up, and explained the play. Vishnu was their friend, it was true, but Vishnu was also the friend of the Asuras - and neither (even together) could have churned the ocean: it was all Vishnu's doing. Shiva explained to them the means of lasting peace, but they were not able to fully understand what Shiva was telling them. Not yet. Shiva grew frustrated - even the Asuras knew what happened, and blamed Vishnu for their misfortune - how could the Devas not understand Vishnu's role in their success?

Shiva also tried to explain to the Asuras that Vishnu was, nevertheless, their friend too, showing them the ways that Vishnu had helped them in the past, and present, the gentleness and kindness shown - and how even the Devas blamed Vishnu for their suffering, and had to have sought Vishnu's help in recovering their vigor and ability of resurrection, how Vishnu had tricked Indra with the bees so that the Asuras could regain their home ... but like the Devas, the Asuras were not quite ready to understand everything Shiva was trying to teach them.

Some beings are able to learn by the simple instructions of Shiva, but others find it necessary to learn by guided experiences, such as the "plays" of Vishnu.

Shiva Purana 21 - Ravana, the mystic

Once Ravana became King of the Rakshasas of Lanka, he performed tapasya to honor Brahma. Dissatisfied with even his extraordinary efforts, having endured constantly day and night, even through the excrement of his own filth, now at the point of despair and madness, he dug a pit on the southern slopes of Himavan, and kindled five fires, giving up his Brahma tapasya, and installing a Siva Linga before him. Ravana then began to cut off his heads (he had ten of them) and one by one sacrificed them in the fire.

At the moment he would have killed himself by cutting off his last head, Shiva Sankara was so disturbed by this that he woke from his meditation and appeared before Ravana. Like a doctor, Shiva aided body and mind: he gently restored the severed heads, and thinking Ravana insane, and that he might similarly relieve Ravana's mental injury, lovingly asked what Ravana could possibly hope for by such self-harm?

Ravana admitted he might be insane, but said, "I love you. I wanted to see you. I want to take this Linga to Lanka, that I may always be as near to you as I am now, that you may always hear me and my people should we require relief. I am now King of the Rakshasas, I want your unequalled strength to protect my people and myself against the Devas, Asuras, Nagas, animals... [he listed every type of being, but forgot to include humans, since he did not fear them - Shiva didn't correct the mistake, as it was clear that Ravana had more to fear from himself than from humans, or anyone else for that matter, and Shiva is not in the habit of correcting mistakes]. I fear that my people will never be safe without this."

Shiva shook his head in disbelief: he couldn't understand why Ravana thought this would accomplish these goals, and yet - here Shiva was, before him, ready to give him what he wanted. Shiva had been tricked. Shiva was a annoyed at having been tricked, and disturbed, and would teach Ravana a lesson. "Well, you are now as strong as you imagine me to be, Ravana. You may take this Linga, Rakshasa," said Shiva, smiling. "But remember - it will remain wherever you set it down first. Don't hand it to anyone along the way to hold for you, and do not set it down until you get to Lanka. Only you can carry it, and only this once."

Shiva went away again and Ravana was so happy. Having bathed and refreshed himself a little, he began. He found he was able to lift the Shiva Linga with no effort at all! He began the long journey back to Lanka. But on the way, that Rakshasa, that master of tapasya, who endured the excrement of his own filth and even cut off his own heads, now felt the need to defecate and decided to relieve himself of this discomfort: the Devas, jealous of Shiva's great gifts, had feared Ravana would use it to attack them, and asked Vishnu for help. Vishnu suggested Varuna to fill Ravana's bowels and bladder with fluid.

At this very moment when he was filled with fluid, Ravana met a cowboy - the cowboy happened to be Vishnu in disguise. The cowboy made some remarks about how Ravana seemed discomforted, and needed relief - then kindly offered to hold the linga while he relieved himself. So persuasive was the cowboy that Ravana hastily agreed, handing the cowboy the lingam and rushing into the privacy of the bushes. Well, Vishnu had intended to give the lingam to the Devas, but as strong as he was, he could hold the heavy linga only a moment or two. Ravana had imagined Shiva was stronger than Vishnu, after all - and now was as strong as he imagined Shiva was. Well, Ravana was gone more than a half-hour! The cowboy had to put down the linga, and it became immovable from that spot: this jyotirlinga vaidyanatha remains today in that spot (it is named after how Shiva was Ravana's doctor, vaidya, in healing Ravana's decapitation).

Try as Ravana could to move it, he could not. In his extraordinary efforts, Ravana even dented it - but it is still there today, and will always remain there.

Well, Ravana could do nothing to move the stone. So he swore to visit it every day if he could, seeking the relief of Shiva. Many pilgrims still visit the stone today, like Ravana would. Perhaps in visiting it you will gain the same relief as Ravana did? Whether in his daily devotions, or nearby that spot in the bushes. Or afterward, in his failure.

Luckily, Ravana still had the immense strength given to him by Shiva, and came home happy to Lanka, satisfied he could protect his people. When his people saw how strong he was, they celebrated him. They knew they would be safe!

But when the Devas heard of this strength, they grew anxious: even without the lingam, Ravana was now so dangerous. Would the Rakshasas now challenge them in war, as the Asuras had so frequently done? It seemed likely - especially once Ravana discovered they had pre-emptively attacked him with fluid. They decided to take another pre-emptive strike. It was at this time that Narada traveled among the Devas, and heard of Ravana's strength, and the fears of the Devas. He assured the Devas not to worry. It was clear to Narada, at least, that Ravana would not remain always protected by Shiva.

Narada was a friend to everyone, humans, animals, nagas, Devas, Asuras, and Rakshasas too. And more than these, besides. Every kind of being, and every individual being he was a friend to! Narada loved to hear their stories. And, this was one story he had to hear first hand! So soon he departed from the Devas, and went to Lanka to visit Ravana. There, he asked to hear the story of what happened. Ravana, of course, was eager to oblige: as much as Narada liked to hear stories, Ravana liked to tell this one. When Ravana came to the part of the story where he was given limitless strength, Narada asked him what he intended to do with it?

Ravana thought a moment, and said "to thank Shiva, I will celebrate our perpetual safety by conquering every world!" Ravana had learned that the Devas had caused him to drop the linga, and considered he might not be safe while the Devas - or anyone else - remained unconquered.

Narada smiled, apparently the Devas were partially correct in being afraid. But Narada, friend to every being, would not permit Ravana to harm anyone else - let alone everyone else! So Narada conceived of a trick.

"Of course you will," Narada said, knowingly. "And you have Shiva to thank for this strength. But you know, he is so absorbed in his meditation, he might not notice how much you love him, how grateful you are, your victories for his sake, or even if you need him to help you. Besides, you dropped the linga, and in trying to pick it up again dented it - this probably insulted him. Perhaps, you should refresh his memory of your love, and perform another tapasya? Might you not with your great strength lift up Kailasa (on which Shiva sits) and gently set it down again, shouting his praise, and thanking him properly? You should wake Shiva from his meditation again and get his attention! Then you can be sure he will keep his promise, forgives you for dropping the linga, and knows how much you love him! Oh, he will be so pleased!"

Ravana, despite his devotion to and love of Shiva, did not actually understand Shiva enough to know this would greatly annoy Shiva. Ravana did not know what would truly thank Shiva, how to express his love to Shiva, or gain the forgiveness of Shiva. Thus, what Narada proposed seemed wise to Ravana. So Ravana promptly did as Narada proposed.

When Ravana lifted up the mountain, every world shook. Ravana shouted how much he loved Shiva, and how sorry he was, and the noise reverberated through all the worlds. Shiva was indeed awakened from his meditation, and startled, grew angry. In alarm, he turned to Gauri (Shivaa) and asked "what is this? Who shakes my mountain and disturbs me?"

Gauri (Shivaa) was also awakened by this shouting and shaking, but instead of growing angry at the surprise, was giggling. She smiled laughed at the whole thing. Especially at Shiva's reaction. "Don't be alarmed, Shiva - it is merely gratitude from your devotee, Ravana the Rakshasa. Can't you hear his shouting? He is showing you how strong he is, how much he loves you, how sorry he is, and how he relies on you for protection."

But Shiva had already lost his temper, and decided to give Ravana an answer: soon enough Ravana would understand how to properly express his devotion. He would learn self-restraint, and how to properly protect his people: not by war, but by peace. He also grew irritated with Vishnu, and all the Devas who interfered with Ravana's journey to Lanka, leading Ravana to even think that he needed to shake Kailash, or conquer every world. And he was annoyed at Narada - since he liked stories so much, Shiva would give Narada more stories than even he would want to hear. Shiva decided he would teach Ravana - and everyone else - a lesson.

But Ravana was shouting so loudly that he didn't even hear the conversation of Shiva and Gauri, did not notice how angry Shiva was, and never knew to ask forgiveness for disturbing him. Nor could anyone else hear Shiva and Gauri over the ruckus, or notice Shiva's anger in the commotion of Ravana's shaking and shouting. Ravana therefore went back to Lanka, happy, certain that in following Narada's advice he had reminded Shiva of his love. And the Devas were happy, thinking that Narada had tricked Ravana into angering Shiva. He would destroy Ravana.

At the moment Ravana would have returned home, Shiva put his foot down and pinned Ravana under the mountain. Ravana understood Shiva was angry, but really didn't understand why. He sang Shiva's praises for years before Shiva finally let him go. Gauri persuaded Shiva to forgive Ravana, and Shiva did feel bad for losing his temper, and the destruction of

Ravana (Shiva exists without Time, and had already/would already destroy Ravana). So Shiva gave Ravana "the laughter of the moon," Gauri's laughter, a precious sword curved like the moon, or a laughing mouth. Shiva also made him an instrument, a veena, to help him sound better (Ravana was not a melodious singer). "Made him" is a pun, as the instrument was literally made out of Ravana. It was at this time that Shiva gave Ravana his name:

Ravana's name means "screamer," or "loud roaring," referencing the unmelodious singing by which he earned Shiva's forgiveness. It also connotes a sarcastic reference to one who is knowledgeable and aware - of the true, material nature of their environment and self ("yasam ravanam") - as Ravana still did not understand why Shiva was angry.

Ravana is renowned as the author and teacher of astrology, folk medicine, spirituality (as opposed to theology), phonics (opposed to linguistics), politics, and other pseudoscience, and is the epitome of excessive or over-education, someone too clever for their own good. He is the "great brahman," and both knew and liked to sing all the Vedas. Often with the accompaniment of his veena.

Ravana at first tried to welcome peace and friendship with all other beings, even trying to make peace between the Asuras and Devas, equally welcoming their priests to his court. But war broke out eventually, despite Ravana's best efforts (perhaps because of them), and he conquered every world. He was greatly angered at the Devas after his brother, Kuber, insulted him, calling him greedy, materialistic, and stupid (all of which, to be fair, were true allegations – especially considering how Ravana responded to them).

He was doomed to this life of ignorance and fighting, and eventual defeat by Vishnu, because a long time before, Ravana and his brother had been Vishnu's doorkeepers - but that is another story. Some of Ravana's human descendants, and also human inheritors, live in Lanka today.

Kuber - the devotee

Kuber was at one time manifested in the City of Kampilya, where there was a Priest named Yajnadatta: he was a scholar of Vedanta, famous and respected. He invested in his son, Gunanidhi, all his knowledge. But the boy was, in secret, addicted to gambling. Despite all the help of his father, he could not overcome this problem. His mother would frequently bail her son out of debt, but hide the fact from her husband - she was afraid that their son's problem would break his heart. She kept telling her son to reform, but this was not helpful. She kept warning her son of the dangers should his problem be discovered: but he was addicted, and could not stop gambling, even though he knew the dangers of it. When her husband would come home looking for his son, she would lie and say that their son had been studying all day, and so went for a walk - when in fact he was gambling.

When the boy, Gunanidhi, was married, he still did not reform. His mother tried to cut him off, but Gunanidhi then turned to theft. One day, his mother caught him stealing from her - and hid the fact from her husband. To stop him from stealing, his mother began to provide for his debts again: she did not want her son to be a thief. One day, his father saw on a stranger a ring that had been given to him as a gift - he accused the man of theft. But the man explained he had won it in a game, and after a short discussion the boy's father Yajnadatta knew everything. He returned home, and asked his wife: "where is the ring you took from my finger when you massaged my hands yesterday?" His wife said she did not know. "Is it where you put the golden vase we once had? The ivory box? The metal jar? The silver statue?" Yajnadatta explained to his wife that he knew everything now, and how she had been lying to him, and even helping his son steal. He said she was not acting like his wife anymore, she had hurt him, and their son, and told he was divorcing her and left her immediately.

When the boy, Gunanidhi, learned of this, he fled the city for fear of being charged with theft, and arrested. He wandered far. He grew hungrier and hungrier, eventually he could go no further. He sat at the base of a tree and waited for death. He had no idea that it was Shivaratri that day, or that he was very near a temple: but when, at dusk, numerous Yogis came to the spot, carrying sweet foods to offer a stone linga, Gundanidhi followed them to the temple. He would not bring himself to beg, so he merely followed stealthily, plotting how to steal the food. Through the night, the Yogis sang and danced. When at last, the Yogis were exhausted and lay down asleep, Gunanidhi snuck into the Temple, carefully stepping over the sleeping bodies.

The lamp was barely lit, and in the dimness, he couldn't even see the food he desired. So, tearing a bit of his clothing, he added it to the flame as a wick. The fire eagerly consumed the fabric, and a bright light illuminated the entire temple - the Yogis stirred, but were not awakened. However, Gunanidhi was startled, and loudly exclaiming the name of Shiva, he grabbed the food quickly, ran to the door, stumbling over the sleeping Yogis, waking them. He tripped down the stairs, and died.

Gunanidhi was bound hand and foot and taken before Yama's Yamadutas. But at the moment of his trial, Shiva's Ganas appeared. They tried to obstruct the Yamadutas from bringing Gunanidhi to trial, and pleaded on behalf of Gunanidhi. "Let him go, he does not deserve your punishment. He is to be taken to Shivaloka." The Yamadutas naturally respected the Ganas, but were incredulous. "What? Apart from all that he has done against his parents, his society and against Dharma itself, surely you are aware of what he did this night against Shiva? He hasn't done one right thing his entire life. He hasn't gone one day without theft. If this thief has a shred of virtue, let us hear of it. We bet he doesn't. If he does, we will let him go with you."

The Ganas said, "Shiva will vouch for this man. He fasted all Shivaratri day, eating nothing. Though he usually was a thief, he stole nothing that day. He heard the Kortirudra sung by Yogis. On Shivaratri night, he hit the lamp brightly, and said the name of Shiva. It was so bright, not a single shadow could be seen on the Linga! He then woke the sleeping Yogis, who were supposed to have been awake, as he had remained. Can you fault him for any of this?" The Yamadutas had to admit, the man was not entirely without virtue, and had lost the bet. Keeping the terms, they surrendered their prisoner to the Ganas, who took him to Shivaloka.

Shiva had Gunanidhi manifest again as Dama, the son of Arindama, king of Kalinga. Eventually, he ascended to the throne after his father died. He was a devouted Shivabhakti. For whatever reason, he particularly practiced the lighting of lamps. And always kept the temples lit. One day, he went to Kashi, to illuminate his mind. Sitting before a linga, after extraordinary Tapasya, Shiva appeared before him, and said, "ask any gift."

Shiva was so bright that Dama couldn't see him. He said, "let me see you without blinking, no gift is greater." When Shiva corrected his vision, Dama looked up and - saw Parvati. He squinted at her, and jealous, muttered to himself - who is this beautiful woman, what tapasya did she perform more perfect than mine? She is lucky to be so near to Shiva. She makes my Tapasya shine." He circled and snarled, and annoyed Parvati. She asked Shiva, who is this Yogi that squints enviously at me and mutters 'you make my tapasya shine?'"

Shiva laughed, "Parvati, it is your son. That's just his way - he isn't malicious, just praising you the only way he knows how." Shiva blessed Dama, saying "you shall be the master of the mountain city of Alaka, you shall be the lord of Yakshas and Guhyakas, king of the Ashvamukha Kinnaras, you shall be the King of all humans, you shall be the guardian of treasures. Gunanidhi, this is your mother Uma - now, take her blessing too."

Gunanidhi laid himself at Parvati's feet. Parvati looked deep within him, and saw Shiva was correct - his jealousy was not malicious, it was simply the limit of his ability to admire. She approached him to embrace him, but though Dama's eyes had been corrected to see Shiva, Parvati was brighter - and when she came close, he was blinded in his left eye, his body was broken and twisted by the light. Parvati withdrew when she saw her nearness harmed him - and understood the reason for his jealousy, his limitation, he was not strong enough to be nearer to her. "Because you are blind in one eye, we will call you Ekapinga (one-eyed), and Kubera because your body was twisted. It is clear, you will be devoted to Shiva forever: since I cannot, let him come to stay near you, let him be your friend."

Theragatha 3.5

Matangaputta said that on a farm, people will shirk their work by saying it is too cold, or too hot or too late in the evening. Shirking their work, the moment for work passes them by, and they may even miss the proper time for planting or harvesting. But whoever regards cold or heat – or even the growing darkness – as nothing more than grass to plow through won't fail his duties to cultivate his heart. Bear into the plow with your chest!

Week 9

SUMMARY.
Beginner's Class: Introduction to satyagraha and fighting yoga, debate, and conflict resolution. Intermediate Class: Use, weaponization and defense of maya. Subduing hatred. Advanced breathing. The vrtrahatha (victory blow, sacrifice of enmity).

Training methods
- Conventional drilling in methodology: staged sparring, paused frequently for analysis, discussion, and guided (socratic) questions, intent on developing experience with strategy. "What should A do now that B has done this? What will that accomplish? Why is this a good goal? How will this accomplish that goal?"
- Assignments to observe fighting, in courts, or elsewhere
- Control over time to permit pause and reflection before reaction
- Mastery by application of 2nd, 3rd and 4th Jnanas, especially anger and fear control, tolerance, and self-control and self-sacrifice.

Fighting yoga

The practice of Hatha is essentially one of fighting, and the cosmology of Yoga is one of constant struggle and conflict. Just as the disheartened Yogi is not depressed, but merely heartless, just as rest is understood as a different expression of action, peace must be understood not as a distinct state from war, but as a different expression of it. The peaceful yogi is the one who has successfully achieved skill sufficient to fundamentally alter their nature and the nature of their world so as to have no more fighting, and who has become strong enough to withstand all attacks.

The weapons, tactics and objectives of war are varied, but it is in the practice of war that we learn who the truest enemy is - and ultimately understand the means of success.

The war of the doves

In the Brahma Purana, there is told a story of war. On the banks of a river there lived many birds. Among them was a dove, whose name was Anuhrada. His wife's name was Heti. Anuhrada was Yama's grandson. Not far away, there was an owl named Uluka. His wife's name was Uluki. Their entire flock of owls descended from Agni. The owls and doves had become enemies, and were constantly fighting.

To help them in their fight, they asked their Devas for help. The doves asked Yama for help, and were given weapons and help. The owls were given weapons and help from Agni. Thus the two Devas came to be in a war: first by proxy (through aiding the struggle of the doves and owls), then as each Deva was responsible for the harm to the other Deva's family, with each other.

With each intervention by the Devas, as they gave more and more help, the war grew more and more vicious, with strikes resulting in counterstrikes, and even attacks on nests, fledglings and eggs.

Non-combatants were harmed, and entire stretches of the banks of the river were destroyed, involving others in the combat. Additional devas joined the fighting, and the war expanded uncontrollably. Soon, all the world would be burned by war!

At last Yama and Agni understood this folly and intervened one last time. They persuaded the owls and doves to forget their hatred, and live together as friends - as Yama and Agni had.

The place where treaties of peace were agreed to became a place of pilgrimage. Where the doves welcomed friendship with the owls became named Yamya-tirtha; where the owls welcomed friendship with the doves became named Agni-tirtha.

Now, this may seem a childish and simple story - until it is considered just how easily we find ourselves in a similar circumstance, engaged against our own interests, harming ourselves, and those we love. Frequently, a nation finds itself in proxy wars, harming its allies. Siblings, friends, spouses, parents and children - all hurt one another from time to time. The error is made by perpetuating aggression, and permitting its persistence. We senselessly divide ourselves in enmity against those whom we share so much in common.

First understand that your troubles are not wholly of your own making. You have inherited not only your own karma, but the karma of those who have proceeded you, and those who surround you. It is unreasonable to suppose your problems will they be solved entirely through your individual effort.

A single house's fire threatens an entire city. You are not alone - and it is reasonable to expect the entire city to defend a single house. It is reasonable to come to the defense of a single house, even if it is not your own, even if you will never live in it.

Though it is natural to turn inward, and forget the world, to fall asleep, and become alone with our thoughts in the quiet, or worse, to lash out in the dark against the shadows and nightmares we imagine to surround us, learn the lesson of Jnana Yoga. It is by desire that aggression is caused, and by desire aggression is conquered.

Do you desire an end to the fighting? Understanding the means to that end, understanding the reason for the fighting, what has been begun may be brought to satisfactory end. As body is brought by Hatha to bear on body, mind upon mind, the victory against fighting is to be had by fighting.

There is an importance of talking with neighbors, to express that friendship we feel, to remind them of our own presence: trust they will have regretted forgetting you, or not being aware of your need. Or understanding your injury they have caused. And it is important, too, to remind ourselves that our friends are there, that we are not alone - as we might regret forgetting they could help. If we permitted ourselves only to be aware of those who were hurting us, we would think the world a dreadful place. But it is much bigger than that. You are surrounded by friends. And restoring friendship with those who have hurt us is also not beyond reasonable expectation. Any more than it is not unreasonable to expect, upon reaching out, to find yourself surrounded by those friends who were always there.

We share one world, and one community - you are an important part of it. It is natural that everyone would care for your well being, as much as their own. For your interests are the same.

This is why it may be said the very necessity for direct action and intervention indicates a crisis that not only should have been avoided, but whose inflammation may yet be avoided.

This is also why it may be said that it is only by indirect action and non-intervention that things permanently change. The opponent is caused by conditions of environment and circumstance, it is best to treat the disease instead of the symptom: fighting an opponent does nothing to change the state of aggression. But addressing the underlying causes of opposition and conflict will. And this requires, to a great degree, altering our selves.

This is why change is the natural constant and in our interests of peace – permitting it to happen is all that is required of the moment. It is our resistance to change that prolongs our fighting. All change occurs through conditions which, themselves, are conditioned upon more subtle factors that gradually incline toward our interests.

It is impossible to utterly destroy every enemy, or dominate them. But coexistence is possible - by embracing the nature of change.

Such a world of change can be a source of anxiety: ancient alliances are altered, and broken, new ones made; allegiance is unreliable. But understanding all beings seek safety from this changing world reveals opportunities for collaboration with our enemies which might otherwise be obscured by overly-tenacious attachments to senseless opposition.

Arthashastra VII: surrounded by enemies

Every relationship has as one of its elements a degree of opposition, arising out of the distinctness of individuality. This opposition can in either extremity manifest as enmity and hostility or in friendship and alliance: both are expressions of opposition. Because of distinctiveness, because of change, the relationship is inconstant, and inconsistent. The efforts taken to maintain the constancy and consistency of the relationship, together with the efforts to discover the present and anticipate the future nature of the relationship, result in fighting. Thus, to a degree, trust (in the nature of a relationship) and confidence (in its consistency and constancy) are actions against fighting. Thus, to a degree, love, friendship and other bhava is an action against fighting.

Even spouses who dearly love each other will fight. Parents fight with their children, siblings fight. Even a person, whose self-interest is uniquely their own, will sometimes cause themselves harm. Relationships evolve and change, and it is possible for an enemy to become a friend, or a friend to become an enemy. Though this nature of enmity or friendship can be controlled to a degree, the goal of any relationship is not the development of friendship or obstruction of enmity, but one's own peace, security and happiness - which can be accomplished whether at war or at peace, and regardless of the nature of one's neighbors.

Know then, though you are surrounded by enemies and potential enemies, as well as friends and potential friends, but the former need not be avoided nor the latter sought. You must rely on your own strength.

Though there is little to be done to defend yourself against an enemy who is intent upon your harm, and war is unavoidable, it is nevertheless possible to be strong enough to withstand such harm, and recover from any injury. Since you cannot easily grow stronger, ending self-harm is necessarily most prudential and first course of action to be taken. It is no use to have pacified your enemies if you continue to harm yourself.

Technical instruction in debate

The Buddha Gotama introduced a new form of debate, "loading the dice," "the safer bet," "cover all bets" - in the sense that one would bet on both red and black, odds and evens, one must presume that the argument presented is both true and false. Even an absurd argument could be correct under certain circumstances: discovering these limits of truth must become the purpose of argumentation.

For example it may be argued that one is not thirsty after drinking water, therefore water suppresses thirst. The safer bet would be to question when drinking water actually suppress thirst and when it does not to understand why and how. Both argument and counterargument are true: the truth lies somewhere in the middle, where each becomes false.

Consequently, the method of pragmatic debate comes to develop not only a better understanding of the subject, but the reason for the disagreement between proponents and opponents. Why does it matter if one can suppress thirst by water? Is someone thirsty?

Thus, argumentation is made only to develop major and minor premises: there is no necessity to debate inferences, deductions, inductions or undertake any other development of these premises. And necessarily concludes when all premises are conditionally accepted.

This method of debate never develops deconstructive antagonism between proponents and opponents, but on the contrary cultivates constructive respect and friendship. A candle may in fact light the darkness - but only to a small radius around the flame. It is the purpose of argument to further extend this enlightenment.

Arthashastra II, X: weaponization of words

Words may be used for friendship, but there are also four means of fighting which may be undertaken by words: negotiation, persuasion, dissuasion, and attack.

Negotiation is undertaken with five strategies: praise (of the opponent), establishing and building upon mutual relationships (co-ordination, mutual society), establishing and building upon co-operations, identification and discovery of individual and shared interests, and pro-spection of new interests.

Inducing an opponent toward your praise is possible by sharing their values, such as family, character, occupation, conduct, belief, learning, property, etc. Inducing co-ordination is possible by socializing with an opponent within their structures of family, schools, religion, friendships, business, etc. Inducing the help of an opponent is possible by being helpful, necessary and useful to them. Inducing pro-spection of an opponent is possible by proposal and bidding, just as asking and offering induces an opponent toward discovering shared interests or respecting individual interests.

Persuasion is undertaken by offering what is desired or either withholding or preventing against what is feared; dissuasion is undertaken by offering what is feared, or either withholding or preventing/obstructing what is desired. Persuasion is the means of agreement and unification, dissuasion is the means of dissention and fracture.

Attack is undertaken by destruction, deconstruction, harassment, taking or plundering: ideas, value, beliefs, reason, argument, identity, understanding, and other intangibles are formed through words, and remain subject to them.

In using words for friendship or fighting, one must avoid clumsiness, contradiction, repetition, bad grammar, wrong words, wrong connotation, incorrect gender, incorrect number, incorrect time, incorrect casing, poor construction or arrangement, wrong address, and other error. Paragraphs must be divided in suitable places to encourage understanding, and sentences joined into paragraphs to promote understanding. And special attention must be paid to the style: for the opponent's culture, caste, family, social rank, age, learning, occupation, property, character, relationships, as well as the time and place the words will be given and received can bring unintended consequence to words.

Arthashastra III: technical instruction in friendship and bonding

There are many ways in which people come to be bonded (friends, married), and they are all approvable - provided that those who are involved in the marriage are agreeable to it. There are many ways in which people come to be separated, or even divorced, but these necessarily do not require the agreement of everyone involved. The correct manner of conduct during such a separation, or divorce, is dictated by the manner by which the bonding, friendship, marriage was entered into, for termination and suspension of such a relationship is as much a part of the practice as the joining. But there are sometimes laws which must be considered: for sometimes, a kind of marriage or separation or divorce is legally prohibited. However, whether these laws are just, and either can or should be enforced, is a question of justice, not of friendship, marriage, and bonding.

[Marriage being a term convenient to encompass friendship, bonding and "lesser" society, and these other terms being non-inclusive of marriage, marriage will be used from here forward - but understand it as a general term inclusive of all socialization: there is no difference in the nature of bonding between the marriage of spouses, the relationship of monks or nuns cohabitating, or an entire society - except for the intensity, and the various responsibilities of those participating in it. Here it is especially important to reflect that this same bond is borne between those in opposition to each other: a society develops between enemies or combatants which is founded on a mutual relationship. Altering the

relationship from one of antagonism, whether intense or unintense, and the responsibilities of these antagonists to each other, is possible. All relationships evolve and change through Time - Vishnu, Dharma. - Editor]

Women are understood to be the same as men in every way that is important when the formation, dissolution, duties and purpose of marriage is considered. Yet sometimes in marriage the duties of men and women are different, depending on the purpose and type of marriage formed, its purpose, and the agreements of those involved regarding the duties of the marriage.

The choice of whether marriage is undertaken between a man and a woman, between men and women, between a man and women, between a woman and men, between women, or between men, depends on the purposes of the family.

There are many kinds of families which are formed by marriage, and it is for the purpose of forming these kinds of families that these marriages are undertaken. The purposes of family are many. Yet for all kinds, family is essential practice required for development and progress. Therefore, because the manner in which marriage is undertaken dictates the kind of family which will be formed by the union, the purpose of the family should guide the choice in what kind of family to form. Indeed, not every type of marriage, or family, is equally suited to every purpose. And each type of marriage has their purposes, advantages, and disadvantages: the choice of what kind of marriage is undertaken should be guided by the purpose of the intended family.

Separation occurs with the division of the family by distance, death, or sometimes even in accomplishing the purpose of the marriage. Sometimes it is for the purpose of separation that joining is undertaken.

Apart from separation, every marriage is understood to exist for a period of time. Sometimes, those joined will rejoin after the separation, sometimes not: this is determined by the Karma of the individuals, for they will require one type of family or another in their next joining depending on their accomplishments of their prior joining. Sometimes, a such a bond of friendship is formed between those joined that they remain in friendship after the termination, and may even desire to be joined again - but whether this is either possible or appropriate depends on their Karma.

There is frequently the situation where a union is made with the intention of remaining joined indefinitely. But these types of marriages come to an end, anyway.

There are many unions which are formed with the intention of short times, even for a day or a night, or an hour or less.

Yet no matter the term, those who are joined have, however briefly, formed a family and all the consenting parties should agree to and approve of the intended term of the union, and its purpose, and see that it is in conformity with the law. And that the rights of each member is respected in the termination.

There are many conditions upon which a marriage must be dissolved premature to its intended term: for failure of duty, for harm to one or more individuals involved, the inadequacy of one or more members - there are many valid and approvable reasons that the purposes of the marriage might not be possible.

Whether there is compensation owed to one party or another in this dissolution is determined by the manner of marriage, and its terms. And frequently the law. But most joinings result in a sharing of the products of that marriage, either equally, or not so equally.

The duties of marriage differ by the purposes of its making, and the manner by which it is formed, but in every case must be agreed to and approved by all participants. For while marriage is necessarily for the purpose of making family (whatever form that family takes), it is not for the purpose of a household (Grihastha) alone that joining is undertaken. Family is appropriate and necessary to the accomplishment of Brahmacharya, Grihastha, Vanaprastha, and Sannyasa. Indeed, there is no difference between the family of monks, and a family of householders.

Nevertheless, there are numerous types of marriages which are not approvable: these must be dissolved as soon as possible in the manner of a divorce or separation, for the victims have rights to be regarded when they are forced into a marriage, or are incapable (by immaturity, senility, mental illness or other disability) from consenting to the terms of a marriage. Sometimes even those who are otherwise capable of consenting can be forced to marry: by coercion, threat, or even by slavery. These victims too must be compensated.

It is generally agreed upon that when marriage is made by purchase, or a marriage proceeds from material need, it is an approvable marriage. Frequently, the sharing of wealth is a purpose for marriage. Except when the one(s) being married do not benefit directly from the purchase, or did not approve of the terms, this can be construed as a form of slavery, where one or more persons are forced to join with another.

Similarly, it is not a joining when the participant(s) are merely companions, in consortium of friendship, through partnership. Partners, or consorts, while not slaves, are also not family - even if they share in the benefits of the consortium by direct payment or share, even if they have merged their households and families. For, without joining, without union, there can be no separation - and it is both the joining and the separation which constitute the practice of marriage.

Duty of war: preservation of the Dharma

The Arthashastra describes the duty of war as dependent upon the objectives of those making it (their Ashrama), as well as the nature (or castes), of the combatants. But the constant among these variables is a common necessity to defend the Dharma upon which all depend.

It is inappropriate (disadvantageous and unnecessary, undharmic) for members of different castes to fight each other because it is inappropriate for members of one caste to utilize the means of war appropriated to another caste, and such combat would inevitably result in different castes fighting each other when their duties are to serve one another. It is also inappropriate for members of different Ashramas to fight each other because it would be inappropriate for combatants who do not share the same objective to strive with each other. This is is the means by which to avoid violence in war; this is the Ahimsa of War, the only way to peace from war: the Dharma must be preserved, and conflict limited to those whom fighting is appropriate.

Violent war, nevertheless, frequently occurs. Violence may result when any one combatant, out of aggression, desire or ignorance undertakes to fight with a member of a different caste, or a different Ashrama. In these cases, it is appropriate for the several castes and Ashramas to join together in the same objective of repelling the invasion, and restoring the Dharma. It is appropriate for all beings to join in the defense of the aggrieved.

Since contention between the various Ashramas and Varna may not be avoided, it is necessary to understand the means of joining in the battles of a member of a different caste, or Ashrama. This prevents violence, and is the surest means to bringing an end to the invasion: fighting defensively against the invader.

The means (strategy) and implements (weapons) of combat depend upon the objective and nature of the combatant, not their opponent. Successfully altering your own means of combat requires technical skill in many forms of fighting.

A Sudra employs their skills of service in combat. The industriousness of the Vaisya becomes their means of combat. The Kshetriyas utilize their power. The Brahmans utilize their noble and royal nature, their leadership.

Of these four means of warfare, the lowest form (basic form) of warfare is diplomatic (which is the best means for a Brahman), the second-lowest form (next more advanced form) of warfare is forceful (which is the best means for a Kshetriya, especially a "soldier"), the second-highest form (second-to-most advanced form) of warfare is economic (which is the best means for a Vaisya), and the highest form (most advanced) of warfare is disobedience and disruption (which is the best means for a Sudra).

This is the proper form of escalation: if the form of warfare which is appropriate to one's caste cannot achieve the goal, whether in war, or in any Dharmic pursuit, even the pursuit of Kama, the warrior may achieve their goal through a higher form of warfare. Yet if even disobedience and disruption cannot achieve the goal, disobedience and disruption are still required of the warrior, for it is forbidden to submit. It would be more shameful to submit than to fail, even through gross incomptenece.

It is not unlikely that a warrior will be conquered, but it would be shameful only if they denied their opponent the right of victory by failing to defend themselves. There is no shame in being overcome, for there is no cowardice in it.

Understand then the secrets to the most advanced fighting:

Understand that disobedience is the tactic by which a fighter persists in their normal duties and refuses to (does not) undertake anything contrary to their duty.

Understand that disruption is the tactic by which a fighter prevents their opponent from acting contrary to their opponent's duty and requires their opponent to undertake their duty.

It is by both disobedience and disruption that an opponent is returned to their proper caste and Ashrama practice. It is by adhering to duty, to truth and love, that one never harms a friend, or violates one's duty to serve those who rightly demand obedience.

The tactics and secrets of other Ashramas and Varna are subtler, but are as easily learned. It suffices to know that if a different means of warfare is required, the warrior should adopt new Ashrama practices to learn and perfect the duties of the different caste. The warrior who has adequately studied the Dharma, the duties, of the several castes and Ashramas has advantage over the warrior who has not: such a yogi may accomplish their goal with greater success, for they may freely move from Ashrama to Ashrama, freely navigate the castes - and outmaneuver their opponent using more advanced forms of warfare. They will never harm a friend, or themselves, they will never act against their self interests.

This is the secret knowledge of mobility: the commercial service of a Sudra permits an industrial productivity of a Vaisya, the industrial productivity of a Vaisya leads to power. This power is cultivated by splendour, firmness, dexterity, bravery, generosity - as is common among Kshetriyas. This lends itself to the development of a noble and royal nature, the foundation of leadership. Such ennobling when perfected by loyalty leads to a Brahman's serenity, self-restraint, austerity, purity, forgiveness, uprightness, wisdom, knowledge and profound understanding and the ability to refrain from and bring an end to all war by restoring the Dharma.

This is the secret wisdom of Satyagraha.

Arthashastra III, 1: restoration of justice

There are four systems of law. Dharma, Vyavahara, Caritra and Rajasasana: but it is power, and power alone, that is the means to Justice. The very nature of a person, their sacred duty, their Dharma, inspires a concept of justice - but Justice, however well conceived, is subjected in great part to its administration. This power, Vyavahara, is the law that permits trade and business, and is the spirit by which justice is habitually administered. Yet Vyavahara, administration, is subjected to the power of character and honor, Caritra, as an oar is the power that both guides and moves a boat: without character, without honor, any administration of justice is directionless, and weak. And so is Caritra subjected to the power of instruction. For law without the effect of improvement, of self-control, devoid of logic and rationality, results in injustice.

Injustice is a contradiction between the systems of laws. For without logic and rationality, or the effect of improvement and self control, there is a contradiction to the theory of honor; without honor, there is a contradiction to the theory of administration; without administration, there is a contradiction to the theory of justice itself.

It is the objective of any war to restore justice.

It is the first duty of every Hatha Yogi to establish justice prior to practice.

Discovering the Dharma of an opponent

Anticipation of your opponent is important to success: understanding their nature is key to understanding what they capable of, and likely to do.

Because of the occasional necessity and their ability for people to perform different duties, it is important to learn to distinguish the nature of a person from the present expression of it so that discovery may be made of the limits of their abilities: a person can never express a greater nature than they have attained, unless they grow stronger to grow their nature. Since conflict is contradictory to growth, it is unlikely that in a conflict an opponent will grow stronger unless given opportunity to rest and recover and reflect. Never permit your opponent to rest, recover or rest. Endurance wins wars.

Within that expression of nature exists a diversity of skill, and it is important to anticipate the competency of your opponent: just because a woman is a warrior does not mean she has mastered every weapon; just because a man might be a businessman does not mean that he may successfully undertake wholesale, retail, manufacturing, trade, finance, or the very numerous other skills of his nature.

Indeed, though that warrior may live by business, and practice business poorly, she remains capable of wielding weapons - but should that businessman practice business well, and have learned to wield many weapons, until he grows his nature, grows strong enough in body, mind and heart to wield weapons - he will continue to think of weapons in business terms, and fight like a businessman, in a businesslike manner. He will not fight as a warrior does. He lacks power.

Nevertheless, he may yet be a formidable enemy, able to endure and strike with considerable force. He may yet be victorious: the relative strength of an opponent matters as much as their skill.

The diplomat may they may serve as the voice of another, they may negotiate to terms, they may present options, they may lead hand in hand -

each subsequent tactic requires considerable growth, and the mastery of many additional skills.

It suffices to say that knowing your opponent's Dharma is indicates the likeliest choice of tactics.

There are several ways that nature is discovered: a person may become stressed, and thus develop requirement for particular skills or to exhibit particular nature. For example, by requiring a person to fight to the extremity of their ability, you will quickly discover the preferred means by which they engage an enemy: whether by diplomacy, force, economics, or sabotage. Understand stress is caused by fear or hope, and thus inspires action: it is expedient to trick an opponent to reveal themselves, by deception they may fear or hope sufficiently to expose themselves.

Another way nature can be discovered is by intoxication: the subject may become tricked by the numerous skills of Maya to reveal their nature without the necessity of stressing them. Pride and love are effective intoxicants.

Of course, in either situation, the subject may either evade the attempt, or in turn deceive the deceiver. The subject cannot evade discovery by long-association. But like any investigation of their past, their associates and present circumstances, discovery by this means is still unreliable, though: evidence of a person's past can be not only confused, but utterly obscured.

The identity of a person is best discovered, however, by analysis of the person's actions: they are compelled to perform according to the limitations of their Dharma, and will always do so, regardless of the form they present. Analyze the intended and unintended results of a person's effort, as well as their conscious and unconscious efforts, if you would know their nature: whether they facilitate, cultivate, act, or command. Observe what they sacrifice, how, and to whom, if you would know their Teacher. Observe their opposition if you would discover their reason for aggression. And bring an end to it.

Vishnu Purana 1: Only fools remain angry

The Sage Parashar's father, Sakti Maharsi, was murdered and eaten by a Rakshasa (demon) named Rudhir. Rudhir had been a human King, but had been transformed into a demon by Vishwamitra. Yet Sage Parashar grew angry at the Rakshasas. In his anger, he began to systematically destroy every Raksasha, seeking to rid every world of Raksashas. He lit a great sacrificial fire, and presented as an offering every Raksasha he captured or killed. Soon, the Raksashas feared extinction. The Raksashas asked the help of Sage Parashar's grandfather, Vasishtha, and he agreed he would talk to his grandson.

Grandfather told grandson that too much anger was not good. Not all Raksashas could be blamed for his father's death. He instructed his grandson in the nature of Raksashas, their place and necessity to the world, and the good things they sometimes did. He explained that in fact, no Raksasha was responsible for his father's death: his father had earned an untimely death by his war with Vishwamitra. His war with Vishwamitra was perpetuated through every world, across all of time, because each combatant sustained their anger against the other. Grandfather told grandson, "a human being naturally gets angry, but only fools remain angry. Sannyasis should not hold on to anything, but should renounce everything. Sannyasis should not hold onto anger. Shun your anger, Sannyasi. Stop your war against innocent demons. Forgive them, and let go of your anger. Sacrifice your anger, not Raksashas."

Thus convinced by his grandfather's instruction, Sage Parashar extinguished the flame of revenge, stopped his war, and propagated his grandfather's Dharma, teaching anyone the same lesson he himself learned. "A human being always bears the consequences their actions, good and bad. Anger destroys all the results of a Sannyasi's renunciation. This is why Sannyasis shun anger." When he began to teach this, Brahma's son Pulastya arrived on the spot and, presenting him with a copy of the Puranas, and being able to trust him with the knowledge therein, instructed him in it.

Preventing counter-force

Friendship is not won or grown by isolation and disrespect, but by association - and respect. When an opponent is disrespected and isolated, they will seek a more advanced form of warfare than diplomacy and come to believe only force will attain their goals. When an opponent reasons that force is required, they will aggressively bring that force in one of five ways: an attack may be brought upon their leadership, the implements of their force, the means of their strength, symbols of their belief, or upon the opponent directly. These objectives are met by three aggressive forces:

"Harm" is the attempt to destroy or weaken the opponent so that opposition is impossible. But even if an opponent were destroyed, their consent would never be obtained - harm therefore does not achieve the goal. Harm is a form of force. And therefore results in similar counter-force.

"Intimidation" is the attempt to compel obedience of an opponent through fear of harm. Obedience is not consent. This does not achieve the goal. Intimidation is a form of force, and results in counter-force.

"Ridicule" is the attempt to ignore or ridicule an opponent so as to deny or discourage their opposition. Though ignored or ridiculed, the opposition still exists. Ignorance is a form of force and results in counter-force.

These three aggressive forces result in a counter-force known as Resistance; such resistance always results in counter-resistance, more force. Which results in further resistance, more force.

Force, used aggressively or defensively, relies on strength, and strength eventually weakens. It is a mistake to trust to strength, to trust to the use of force, which will ultimately tax your strength. Consequently, a defender will attempt the use of dialogue, reason, debate and similar discourse as non-forceful means of obtaining the consent of an opponent.

A dim candle burning all night long illuminates better a firebomb ever could. A little progress suffices against efforts which are contrary to the goal.

You have greater power of self-harm than your opponent has power to harm you. Not acting contrary to your interests is the wisest course of action.

Arthashastra Book VI: theory of leadership

Leadership is not mystical. There is no divine right of Kings or Republics. There is no natural form of government: societies organize themselves in the means most efficient to their needs and values. Leaders of society naturally arise through inherited intergenerational wealth, of financial, scientific, technical, political and industrial nature. This is mistaken for nobility. Leaders of society naturally arise through honor and reliability, through valor and courage, through reliance on experienced advisors, through personal experience, through honesty, through a cooperative and collaborative nature, through gratefulness and courtesy, through ambition, through enthusiasm, by avoiding procrastination, through self-control, through resolution, through well-skilled servants, through discipline. People will naturally give fealty to such a leader possessed of these qualities.

And when there is but one such leader, an autocrat is seen to arise. When there are a few such leaders, monarchy is seen to arises. When there are more such leaders, a republic arises. When there are many such leaders, a democracy arises.

To dominate or conquer your enemy it is necessary to become their leader; understand not only who their leaders are, but the source of their leadership; become a better leader.

The means of becoming a better leader are simple. To improve your intellect, develop curiosity, inquiry, learning, perception, memory, mental reflection before and after action, deliberation in taking action, logic (especially inference), and decisiveness. Valor, determination, purposefulness, quickness, and probity will all improve enthusiasm. Develop self-control through training, self-improvement, foresight, opportunism, good humor, leniency and mercy, freeing yourself from emotionality, smiling, and maintaining the customs of the elderly.

A well endowed land will produce a leader, or if there is democracy there, a rich people. A well endowed leader is, similarly, an asset to their people. As the highest use of wealth in the treasury is to withstand calamities of long duration, so too is the highest use of the leader to protect their people from fickle luck. Many misfortunes are apt to occur, even in a well-endowed land: war not least of them. Always be prepared for this, and all other emergencies. Not every emergency can be foreseen or prepared for, and sometimes strength and readiness are insufficient - but no leader ever failed for having become too strong, too ready.

A leader who is unprepared and unready, one who is of poor character, unintelligent, or otherwise has become their own enemy is easily uprooted. A leader who may be made to become their own worst enemy is soon destroyed. But a leader who is their own friend will persist, for persistence is part of their nature. Even if one good leader possesses only a small Kingdom, that leader will conquer the world with their leadership, and will never ever be defeated or conquered.

Phases of fighting

When first encountering an aggressive opponent is is necessary to discover what type of aggression motivates them, so that proper defense can be made.

Therefore, before hostilities begin, ask for peace to determine what they ask for. If they ask for things or for homage, you may be certain they are motivated by greed. If they are motivated by Justice, they will demand duty, correct behavior, or the restitution of wrong. If they are motivated by hatred, they may pretend toward either of these, or demand nothing at all. Yet the hateful enemy will not come to terms of peace. It is right and honorable to purchase peace so long as the cost of peace is less than that of war, and is not unbearable to the point of representing injuries which cannot be recovered from. This is dharmic.

It is right to seek the adjudication and mediation of a disinterested third party if it is doubtful whether such a peace would be honorable.

But it is never right to submit to hatred: it is impossible to make peace with hatred, anyhow.

The first phase of warfare therefore is the attempt for peace. Should peace fail, the second phase is understood to be an act of rebellion: all self-defense is an act of repelling one who would dominate you, and understanding that you are rebelling against them (rather than they are rebelling against you) is a necessary perspective for success. The goal is the restoration of peace, justice and wealth - not the destruction or domination of the former aggressor. Aggression need not lead to further aggression. Nor should not.

No enemy may be made harmless, but the cost of peace may be reduced so that it is not onerous or infamous.

Sacrifice of enmity, the victory blow: vrtrahatha

The vow for which fighting was begun must be fulfilled before the weapons of that war may be sacrificed. The blow or force which brings final victory in battle (the Vrtrahatha) is the one which fulfills the vow (Vrata) which was made upon bringing or meeting conflict. It is the total destruction (sacrifice, slaying) of enemies (Vrtra). As the cloud builds potential for rain and thunder to emerge from it, and upon releasing these dissipates, so does fighting (from the moment of the vow beginning the war) build potential for its own ending.

It is the blow or force which brings peace, which restores justice, which brings final victory in battle. Though commonly misunderstood to be an honorable act of murder (or suicide) - for the word does imply the killing of enemies - it more accurately may be rendered as "the ending of hostility." Killing an enemy has never resulted in peace: but a sacrifice of enmity has.

Vrata is an act of abstinence which is conducive to continence, it is an act of self-restraint.

Commonly, a little blood suffices to satisfy the human ambition for wrath. Humans are typically content to slay or torture each other on an individual basis. Yet there may come a time of mass intoxication, when in anger numerous people gather for the purpose of a mele, and organizing themselves into battalions exhibit the most exquisite form of hatred, one which cares nothing for the consequence of war, and forgetting even the reason that the war was begun, neglect to understand that in the intoxication of anger no vow was made to consecrate the fighting. Such a drunkard does not know when to stop their fighting. For such a drunkard, there can be no Vrthahatha. Such a drunkard is easily conquered by the Vrata of the conqueror.

Before engaging an opponent in any conflict, whether economic, spiritual or martial, be sober, self-restrained and fully aware; become a soldier of Peace if you desire victory. Peace will always win - in the end. Know when to stop. Yoke yourself to your vow.

Indra's Vrtrahatha

In one particularly dramatized battle against Vritra (Vrtra), Indra is depicted as fighting an enemy whose weapons were Maya, with his own weapons of Maya. Indra and Vritra were equally matched, the two were consumed by the other's weapons and it took Saraswati to discern the victor: she was able to understand the intention of the deception, illusion and delusion cast by each magician by comprehending not only its ultimate (final) result, but also its ultimate (first or primordial) cause. When she revealed these ultimate conditional causes and conditions, she broke the spells of Maya cast by both combatants, and a truce was agreed upon: though nuanced and complex, it may be summarized to say that Indra's enemy fought for hatred and revenge, both of which are self-defeating cause - whereas Indra fought for mercy and self-preservation. Though Indra had done a great wrong, his enemy did a greater wrong through acts of hatred and revenge which harmed not only his enemy, but the entire world as well. After the truce, the two combatants ended up fighting again. But because Indra had kept the terms of the truce, Saraswati used Maya to appear like Indra, and standing beside Indra to defend Indra, defended him.

Durga puja: a puja for weapons

Venerate with Pujas weapons, tools, instruments, even pens and pencils, anything which you use for your work - because they are the means by which you subdue hatred, desire and fear, and shall become victorious against injustice, ignorance and evil. What is an painter without their brush? What is a warrior without their knife? Though one cannot kill, both are weapons against hatred.

This is why we must use the correct tools, and use the correct tools correctly: just as some weapons are cruel, such as barbed or poisoned arrows, even a pencil can be misused to inspire fear, desire or hatred. This is why we should fight ethically, non-violently, in Satyagraha.

Sutta Nipata 4.15: Sacrifice of weapons

The Buddha Gotama said, there is no security or safety from arming one's self, only fear. If arming one's self protected one from attack, or aided in one's defense, there would not be so many people presently fighting each other, having fought each other for so long. Hostility is the cause of fighting, or insecurity, of weapon-taking. Like a painful sting or thorn whose pain causes a person to run about and rave insanely, only when hostility is taken out is there an opportunity to settle down; only when hostility is removed is there an opportunity for peace. To remove hostility, one must no longer grieve, one must no longer mourn. To become beyond grief, beyond mourning, you must become dis-attached, let go of the past, and sacrifice all that is yours. All that has gone before. And all that is to come - have no hope for it. Have no fear of it. Courage! In sacrificing your weapon, in sacrificing your safety, in sacrificing everything.

[Editor's note: the weapon which is not sacrificed will eventually result in self-harm. Understanding the appropriate time and manner of the sacrifice

is less important than the actual practice: generally, the sacrifice is made after puja. Whether early, or late, the sacrifice itself will be successful, for it forces the sacrificer to understand the reason weapons were taken up in the first place. Consider, too, there are many forms of weapons: economic, political and diplomatic weapons can both be injurious and deadly - even an empty hand is a potent weapon, as it will not stay empty long]

Technical instruction in the weaponization and defense of maya

Deception, illusion and delusion (Maya) are broken (sacrificed, given up) by a process of analysis which categorizes the phenomenon or form of Maya into its elemental components and conditional components. This is symbolically represented by a rainbow, which is an illusion: when it is analyzed, the rainbow is seen to be the result of many droplets of water prismatically reflecting, refracting and dispersing sunlight. When the cause and components of the illusion are known, the illusionary rainbow ceases to deceive the eye into delusion. Similar rainbows, formed by the prismatic nature of glass or diamonds, can even be reconstructed into integral white light by returning, de-refracting, focusing the light.

The rainbow is associated with Indra, a Deva whose tools include a diamond - symbolizing this ability to break deception, illusion and delusion, and which also controls rainbows. This diamond takes the form of a weapon, specifically a lightning bolt, instantaneously and violently breaking Maya. It is interesting to notice, as well, that the process of breaking Maya is identical to the process of weaving it: this is further symbolized in the other tool of Indra, the rainbow (depicted as a kind of net that both ensnares, as a typical net would, and propels missiles, as a typical bow would) - and how Indra fights both with weaponized Maya and against weaponized Maya.

The Arthaveda describes how to create and use these tools and use them, as well as how to weaponize Maya, to protect against fraud, deceit and criminals. These tools (and weapons) are also described in special application within the Kamashastras. And in other documents as well. In every Ashramic practice, it is necessary to understand not only how to break deception, illusion and delusion - but how to use them, as well, for the purpose of bringing an end to distress, the dangers of using them wrongly - and training rules for how to avoid wrong use.

Maya is an important and necessary tool for practice: beside permitting understanding of what is abstract by giving form to formless constructs (drawing a circle is impossible, but a close rendering using maya permits even advanced practices of geometry; graphical representations of numerical data are also maya, as are maps, etc. and also stories, like the puranas, and plays and games), beside permitting communication and interaction and instruction, maya is the best means of self-control.

Illusion is absolutely necessary for constructing abstractions which represent real phenomenon in ways more suitable to analysis, delusion is often helpful in understanding different perspectives, even deception is sometimes necessary to save a life. It is necessary in war, and peace. Would you use Maya as a defensive weapon and lie, saying you do not know where someone is, to save their life - or even conceal them from their enemies? Would you pretend to be someone else other than who you are to save them, as Saraswati rescued Indra? Would you pretend to a different identity to "walk a mile in their shoes" act as a more loyal agent in a business deal? Would you construct elaborate illustrations and diagrams to understand geography, or astronomy? There is good reason to rightly do these things, to rightly use Maya. But for the purposes of fraud, to perpetrate acts of hatred and harm, Maya (whether a tool or a weapon) becomes self-destructive, and self-defeating - and cannot obtain the goal for which it is purposed.

Technical instruction in controlling Time and Dharma

While speedy reaction is conducive to success, premature reaction is contrary to success. It is important to not react blindly or automatically, but to consider carefully each response. But not for so long that the opportunity for action fades. In any fighting, whether a physical fight or a verbal fight, emotionality may take over when the feeling of urgency (being rushed or being injured and out of control) is experienced.

Maya is an important tool for the fighter: controlling the perception of time is useful. Sometimes time may seem to pass too quickly, or too slowly. Generally, heightened awareness or concentration in any of the jnanas permits control over the perception of time: it is by distraction and lack of awareness that pain lends an illusion of slow-time, and pleasure lends an illusion of fast-time. Beyond pleasure and pain, time is perceived very differently, and sometimes not at all.

Fear of injury or anger, or other anxiety, may heighten the sense of pain, and cause time to move out of control. It is sometimes helpful to maintain the perspective that whatever injury is experienced is typically not beyond the ability to recover from, and practice jnana yoga: awareness of body and mind, especially, to understand this pain, injury, fear and anger, so that control may be maintained. Having sacrificed attachments to body and mind, when either are injured, the lack of attachment will permit greater freedom in response: it will be possible to "roll with the punches," or to permit injury knowing you are strong enough to withstand it, and recover.

It may also be helpful to practice the bhavas, or at least honor your opponent. Puja for your opponent or your weapons will cultivate confidence and love. Feel love and compassion for your opponent, feel compassion and love for your tools. Respect them, and see you are worthy of your opponent and your weapons.

Stay aware of how the opponent was not always in a state of aggression, and will not always remain aggressive. Understand their vow. Being aware of your own body and mind, extend your awareness to encompass theirs. Understand the nature and causes of the conflict, remember the vows made by both you and your opponent, and acting as Priest for both yourself and your opponent, perform the vrtrahatha, and ensure your opponent's successful vrtrahatha as well.

If your opponent is crazed, or utterly irrational, if there has been no vow, in short, if Self-defense is required, having performed the self-sacrifice, it will be easier to defend your Self for the sake of all those who depend on your Self, rather than fall into the rush of emotionality resulting from attachment to self. Then, you will act with the minimum violence to prevent harm to yourself or others and may in fact assist your opponent in their recovery, or at least prevent them from causing regrettable harm.

It may seem impossible, but it is always possible to pause, even for a split second, during a conflict. In this pause, you will be able to think with clarity, and extend that moment into sufficient time to consider options for success. One of the best ways to pause is by breathing once, perceiving the heartbeat, or the body: this short-cut to the first jnana is helpful in attaining greater jnanas.

Bear in mind it is not necessary to act on emotions, sensations, or thoughts which are experienced. Rationally consider your options.

Ultimately, the best advice is practice and observation. Being curious about fighting, observe those engaged in combat, whether in the courts, their businesses, their homes, or elsewhere. Familiarity removes the unknown, which can reduce the fear of the fight: the harm we anticipate from the fighting is often worse than the harm that we are actually likely to experience. Understanding the means and necessity for reconciliation permits contemplating how any action taken during the fight may expedite this goal.

Fighting may be unavoidable, and loss of control is also likely. However, the fighter who regains control quickly may prevent an escalation of fighting, and speed the resolution of the conflict.

Breath

A breathing technique which is good to practice is pausing between breaths: pausing before breathing in and pausing before breathing out. This stills the mind, and permits it to calm. It also presents an opportunity for meditation in that moment between breath.

The monk, Rahula, Gotama's son, once asked what to meditate on while breathing. He was told:

"In practicing breathing meditation, a monk will go into the wilderness to the shade of a tree, or into an empty building, sitting down, mindful of his breathing in, and breathing out. Breathing in, he discerns, 'I am breathing in.' Breathing out, he discerns 'I am breathing out.' If he breathes deeply, he discerns that. If he breathes shallowly, he discerns that. By his breathing, he discerns his entire body, its organs, its tissues, its fluids, its air, its wastes, even his mind. He understands the nature of his form, his feeling, his perception, his imagination, his consciousness. He calms his attachment to his form. He steadies and satisfies his mind, releasing it. He develops good will, and abandons ill will; he develops compassion, and abandons cruelty; he develops appreciation, and abandons resentment; he develops equanimity, and abandons irritation; he becomes aware of beauty, and abandons his desire; he becomes aware of inconstancy, and abandons his conceit of 'I am.' Breathe in and out, and be aware of your breathing, your body, its numerous tissues and organs, its form, and the form of the air you are breathing, and the form of the world in which you are sitting. Breathe in and out, and understand, whatever is subject to origination is all subject to cessation."

"The form of your body is not yourself. Neither is the form of your world, nor the form of your work, your clothes, your other possessions, your home, nor any other form you take. Neither are your emotions yourself. Neither are your perceptions and beliefs yourself. Neither are your thoughts self. Neither is your consciousness yourself."

Interrupting breath

Gotama taught many methods of meditation. One was a meditation of interruption as a means for developing the awareness required for freedom from suffering. The interruption takes the form of a breath.

Gotama said this meditation should be undertaken in the wilderness, or at the foot of a tree in a park, in an abandoned building, or even amid the trash and filth of a city – while sitting, standing, or walking, while falling asleep, waking up, talking or remaining silent, while when eating, drinking, chewing and tasting, even when urinating and defecating. It should be undertaken frequently, anywhere and at any time.

Taking a breath in and out, become aware of your bodily actions at that moment. If you are sitting, become aware that you are sitting. If you are standing or walking, become aware that you are standing or walking. This is done, whatever it is you are doing, by taking a breath in, and a breath out, and doing nothing for that moment – and recognizing by that interruption what you had been doing.

With another breath in and out, recognize what you were thinking – all the things you anticipated happening if you interrupted, or didn't interrupt, all the things you were preoccupied with. Recognize what you were feeling, emotionally with your mind and sensually with your body, the pleasure, the pain – and your instinctual pursuit of pleasure and avoidance of pain. Become aware of all your habits and instincts - and recognizing that they may be interrupted.

With another breath in and out, recognize that they may not only be interrupted, but abandoned.

With another breath, become aware of your choices to continue your behaviors, or assume new ones, and cultivate the purpose of rationality, logicality, of acting rightly without regard to instinct or habit.

With another breath, recognize that action is not necessary at this very moment of interruption, of stillness, of doing nothing.

Now that you are interrupted, with another breath in and out, become aware that you are breathing. Become aware of all that your body is doing, even when stilled. Study your body, study your mind.

Breathing in and out, study your body, recognize, as a butcher would examine a carcass, as a scientist would study an animal, that there hairs on your body, nails, teeth, skin, muscles, tendons, bones, bone marrow, kidneys, heart, liver, spleen, lungs, large intestines, small intestines, a colon, feces in that colon, bile, phlegm, pus, blood, sweat, fat, tears, skin-oil, saliva, mucus, fluid in the joints, urine – all the different components of your body. These are all sustained through breathing.

Breathing in and out, recognize that they are sustained through eating, drinking, working, exercising – all the actions you require to survive.

Breathing in and out, recognize that you were born only by your father and mother sustaining themselves, and sustaining you. Recognize the endless sustenance which they required – from their parents, and their parents' parents.

Breathing in and out, recognize you will grow old and die – even if provided with adequate sustenance. It is inevitable that you will die, your body will bloat and become fetid and festering, and eventually decompose.

Breathing in and out, recognize you will become sick and grow weaker with age – even if provided with adequate sustenance. This is inevitable.

Breathing in and out, recognize your present strength, your present life, your present breathing.

Breathing in and out, become aware of your mind – each thought, each memory, each belief requires sustenance. As does each emotion. These are also impermanent, changing. They can be let go of.

Now, aware of your body, breathe in and out, and interrupt that sustenance – if only for a moment. Become calm, composed, still, without pleasure or pain. Become equanimous, mindful and alert - if only for a moment.

In this moment of neither pleasure nor pain, no-thought, no-action, become aware that you are without suffering – and become aware of how suffering arises, and how it ceases.

Conquer both your displeasure and your delight. Conquer fear and dread. Resist cold, heat, hunger, thirst, the touch of flies and mosquitoes; resist the wind, sun, and every creeping thing. Resist abusive, hurtful language. Cultivate endurance of bodily and mental feelings that, when they arise, are painful, sharp, stabbing, fierce, distasteful, disagreeable, deadly.

Develop your ability to – at will, without trouble or difficulty – interrupt your behaviors, master your habits and instincts. Develop your constant awareness of your actions of mind and body, remain purposed in your heart toward rightness.

Let go of your beliefs – even those beliefs of impossibility. Impossibility is just a belief, too – perfect your knowledge of how things are. You are neither one nor many, you are neither here nor there, walls and mountains present no obstacle, the earth itself is like water, water is like dry land, you can fly through the air, and even touch the moon and sun.

Cultivate your hearing, your sight, all your perception, purifying them through greater attention. And with this perception and attention become aware of the minds of others, their suffering, their avoidance of pain, their seeking pleasure, their ignorance, their hate, their habits, their beliefs, their impossibilities and possibilities, understand their minds.

Understand your changing being, your self, your many lives - even within this same body. Study them, the birth, the sustenance, the death. What you did, what you didn't do – and why. See the many lives, the many becomings and endings of all beings, understand the cycle of birth and death, of rebirth and redeath, the consequences of actions both good and bad. And the advantages of non-action.

End your suffering.

Anguttara Nikaya 5.162: subduing hatred

Sariputta said hatred should be subdued. These are five ways of subduing hatred.

There is the hatred which arises when observing impurities and imperfection. When a person is impure in their actions but pure in their words, or pure in their actions but impure in their words, how should such hatred be subdued?

It is as if you dropped a rag in the road, half in a puddle: you would tear off the sound part and continue along the road with it. In the same way, pay no attention to the impurity observed, instead pay attention only to the purity observed.

Or it is as if you were traveling and became thirsty, overcome with heat, covered with sweat, exhausted, trembling with dehydration and you had found a pool of water overgrown with slime. You would part the slime and then drink from the pure water underneath and continue along your way.

Sometimes hatred arises because a person is periodically clear and calm and pure in both words and actions, but usually isn't. How should such hatred be subdued?

It is as if you were traveling, thirsty, dehydrated – but instead of a pool with slime, you came upon a cow footprint filled with water. Trying to drink from it, you would disturb the water and make it unfit to drink – so you would have to get down on all fours and slurp it. So should you pay close attention to the times of clarity and calm, the momentary purity.

There are some people who are always impure in action and word, who never experience clarity and calm. How should hatred be subdued for them? It is as if you found a sick man, seriously ill and in pain, along a road, far between any place of help, unable to eat, unable to get medicine, unable to drink, entirely alone without assistance. In compassion, you would try to help that man, and if you couldn't carry him to help, you would carry food, water, medicine and other necessary help even a long distance to help him.

So should you help the man who is impure in both action and body, and without even momentary clarity and calm.

Sometimes, too, you may see a person who is pure in both action and word, and yet sometimes imperfectly loses their mental clarity and calm. How do you subdue hatred for them? It is as if you found a pool of clear water – sweet, cool, limpid, with gently sloping banks, shaded on all sides with trees of many kinds – and you had come along, burning with heat, exhausted, trembling with thirst. Having bathed in the pool and drank from it, you would rest yourself in the shade of the trees. It would not matter to you that sometimes the pool is disturbed. So should you, when they lose their clarity and calm, pay attention to their purity of action and word.

Against hatred, make the mind grow serene.

Sutta Nipata 1.7: Outcast/Outcaste

When Gotama was living near Savatthi at Jetavana at Anathapindika's monastery, he had entered the City for alms. At that time, a Brahman, Aggikabharadvaja, who was notorious for his strict religious observance, was conducting a fire sacrifice. When the Brahman saw Gotama, he became terrified that his sacrifice would be ruined: Gotama was an outcaste: he had no caste, for he had been born into one one caste, then gave up all caste, adopting the duties of all the others. Having no caste, no society, he had no duty - and violated the Dharma of Vishnu, whom the Brahman was now honoring.

"Get away!" shouted the Brahman, almost hysterically. "Go! You shaved your head, but you are a wretched monk! You are an outcast - an outcaste!"

Gotama replied calmly to the Brahman, "do you know, Brahman, what an outcast is, and what makes an outcaste? It would be good if you'd permit me to explain the Dharma, as you are yourself rejecting the duties of your caste, and will be cast out by the members of your caste." The Brahman calmed for a moment, and asked Gotama to explain. Gotama then explained,

Not by birth is one a Brahman, by self-control alone one becomes a Brahman. By lack of self-control one becomes an outcaste.

Caste, society, is not given by birth. Nor are the duties of that society.

A true outcast, a true outcaste, a true criminal has no good society, no good friends - for they are not a good friend, nor good to associate with. They have both rejected their duty, and been turned away by those who would perform their duty.

They are angry. They shelter and protect their hatred and distaste, reluctant to speak well of others, discredit the good in others, they are perverted in their views and deceitful. If asked to say something good, they say what is detrimental, or talk evasively.

They will needlessly kill living beings, whether born of womb, egg or seed without regret, they have no sympathy for living beings. They are not worthy of the honor their food does them.

They terrorize their village or city, and become notorious as an oppressor.

Whoever takes what is not given to them is an outcast, an outcaste. They have no good society, no good friends - for they are not a good friend, nor good to associate with. They have both rejected their duty, and been turned away by those who would perform their duty.

Having incurred a debt, they run away when pressed to pay, saying "I owe you no debt!" They do not acknowledge all that conditioned their own success.

Desiring something, they kill or weaken the person in possession of that thing, and grab what they desire - or make lies to obtain what they desire. They will lie for the purpose of deception itself - or to obtain what they want. Or merely to hurt, and deprive someone else of what they cannot have.

By force or by consent, they sexually associate with the spouses of relatives or friends, and others whom they shouldn't.

Being wealthy, strong, able, or youthful, they do not support their parents when their parents are growing old.

They strike or hurt by words their family and friends.

They would try to commit a wrong action in secret, so that it may not be known by others - not understanding the nature of truth, that it cannot be hidden, they do not understand the necessity for it, either.

They will go to another's house, enjoy choice foods, and then not return the honor to their host by equal hospitality when their host repays the visit.

They are like a beggar who appears at mealtime with harsh words, or like a person who would not offer a beggar food.

They exalt themselves by belittling others, they are selfish, shameless. They have no fear of the consequences of their bad actions.

They revile the Buddhas, they revile householders (Grihasthis), they revile recluses (Sannyasis).

They pretend to be a Buddha, a householder, or a recluse - when they are not one. And this is the worst sort of criminal.

When Gotama said this, Aggikabharadvaja thanked him, "just as a man were to set upright what had been overturned, or reveal what had been hidden, or point the way to one who had gone astray, to hold an oil lamp in the dark for someone else to see things, in this way, you have shown me the Dharma. I take refuge in the Buddha Gotama, his Dharma and his Sangha. May Gotama accept me as one of his students!"

Rig Veda Book 6 Hymn 75

See? Barbed arrows dipped in poison already fly at you, falling about you like hair at a barber's. Do not suffer their offense further: hurry into battle, meet your opponent closely, strike your opponent before they kill you!

Defend that life your parents gave to you with the strength they gave you to defend it! All those who love you call you to battle, that you may not be dominated by your opponent's hatred; it is for love they ask you to rush into battle, that you may be victorious, with unwounded body.

Even your opponent calls you into battle!

Eagerly seek this battle!

Trust to your strength and life. Trust to the thickness of your armor to protect you. Trust your horse; it has always been free, like your heart's will. It shall faithfully carry you to meet your enemy. Because of its nature, its love and its duty, it shall not flinch at the opportunity to defend you by trampling and crushing your enemy - do not you hesitate a moment! You are so admirably armed: trust to your weapons to turn the hatred of your opponent to grief and sorrow.

Have no doubt: you shall be victorious and subdue their hatred!

Week 10

SUMMARY.
Beginner's Class: Purpose of practice. Introduction to performance. Purpose of life. Intermediate Class: Begging. Recycling. Waste. Sacrificing honor and dana. Perversion. Priesthood. Vishnu. Laxmi.

Training methods
- Practice in emulation
- Practice in creation
- Practice in giving
- Practice in begging
- Recycle old cloth, or other waste items
- Practice in spring cleaning

Purpose of practice

Performance in the context of duty is best understood through the performance arts, and especially the natya shastra. Though, of course, like all shastras, modern technology and technique far exceeds ancient methods, the theory of performance remains virtually unchanged, practicable and useful to learn.

Succinctly, the purpose of practice is performance. It is by the performance arts the Dharma, the Avatar of Vishnu, is manifested and communicated.

Introduction to performance: Natya Shastra

While entertainment is a desired effect of performance arts, it is not the primary goal. The performance arts remains the very best method by the Dharma, the Avatar of Vishnu, is manifested and communicated. Such Natya Shastra (representation of acts; Acting) is often the only means by which a student may come to understand the Dharma.

Performance arts includes acting, music, fashion, architecture, engineering, writing, sciences, and the performance of all other arts. The performer (no matter their art) is best described as an "actor," though the term has come to be associated only with the dramatic arts.

Natya Shastra has two fundamentals: emulation and creation.

Emulation. An Actor will study the dharma, which can be best learned through the artistic performances of others. After sufficient study, the actor will manifest by Maya (magic, formation) a representation, reproduction, or example of the subject they have studied.

Creation. The Actor who has sufficiently studied their art will come to understand the Dharma. Then, by Siddhi, they will manifest the Dharma, first within themselves, then within their audience.

In the Samyutta Nikaya 42.2, the Buddha Gotama describes a very real danger actors face. Maya is a dangerous weapon, as it is easy to inflict self-harm.

Creative Siddhi is permitted (appropriate) only under very specific and limited conditions: it is frequently far better to provide emulation of the Dharma. It is usually important that an audience come to discover the Dharma themselves, for there is much benefit in the process that transmission by Siddhi would rob them of.

Priesthood. In those circumstances when Siddhi is required, the Actor should first inspire joy through the several skills of leadership: when the audience takes joy in the act of communicating, their insight will be heightened sufficiently to themselves perform (Dharmi) their duty, to achieve their nature, to embody the Dharma. Thus, the Actor performs (Dharmi) both the duty of the audience and themselves, as if the audience were an instrument or clay, shaped into the necessary form. In this function, the actor is performing as a Priest.

When is Siddhi required? When the audience is incapable of understanding the Dharma if it were merely communicated through emulation (such as because of inexperience, disbelief (unbreakable religious faith), doubt, physical or mental deficiency, profound emotionality, constraint or imprisonment or other lack of freedom such as addiction, etc.).

The Bridle

The concept of taming one's self is often translated through the imagery of a tamed horse or ox - one which can wear a bridle (Yama) is evidently at least somewhat tamed. Yamas (and Niyamas) are evidences of this gentleness, which in English has the similar double meaning of nobility. This is part of the reason it is said, with double meaning, only a devotee of Vishnu can master Yama, can hold their own bridle.

Purpose of life

Work is a means of life in Grihastha and Vanaprastha. Jiva is a word that means "condition of life" or "manner of life." A coppersmith is a tamrajiva: copper is their life. Grain, the basis of human diet, is jivanarha. When life ends (jivananta), it is understood that the conditions for living have ended, in the sense that a candle is extinguished when deprived of oxygen, wax fuel, or wick to carry wax to the air in fueling combustion. Work is the means by which Yoga is performed - and perfected. It is the purpose of life.

Sacrificing Dana and Honor

Dana is a concept of not withholding what is not yours, or, alternatively, what is someone else's. In a practice of sacrifice, what is not yours you cannot sacrifice. You cannot give what is not yours. You cannot use it up, or destroy it. You cannot attach to it, nor detach from it. You cannot renounce it.

That which has been entrusted to you is the property of another, but the duty is still yours.

The practice of sacrificing dana, of holding onto what is not yours, is different from the practices of acquisition, from Artha.

Enemies exchange their hostility for dana, love and friendship grows through dana. Consider your opponent: what do they hold that is yours? Consider your duty to take what is held wrongly from you. Practicing the yoga of fighting, discover the opportunity to sacrifice all that is yours for an end to conflict. Consider who holds your heart, and how you might be worthy of theirs.

The sacrifice of dana begins by understanding the nature of self, what is yours, through jnana yoga. The Buddha taught that whoever discovers the nature of self through jnana yoga will regard all their forms, past, present or future, internal or external, coarse or fine, lofty or low, far or near, any form at all they should regard as not theirs, not what they are, not their Self. Therefore, they also regard their emotions, perceptions, thoughts and consciousness thus: 'this is not mine, this I am not, this is not my self.'"

The beggar, in asking dana, is asking for what is their own, and asking what does not belong to the donor. The beggar has a duty to help the giver understand their self, and overcome their attachments.

The giver has a duty to evaluate if what is being asked for is their own.

Merely providing food or money or other necessities to another is not dana, but it can be an act of dana. It is not sacrifice, but it can be an act of sacrifice. It may or may not be appropriate or useful.

When does a person have nothing left of their own to give? At such a point, they are ready to sacrifice dana. At such a point, they have already sacrificed all honor. At such a point, they are prepared to gain, to acquire, ready for Artha, to gain honor, and many other things besides.

Introduction to begging

Gifts, or donations, must be given, freely and for the right reasons. The purpose of begging, then, is not merely to raise the material requirements of food, medicine, money, or other necessities. The beggar who would become a conduit of donations (simply conveying the donations to a receiver) fails.

No matter how wholesome and healthy the food is that may be donated, it will soon be turned into excrement and urine. No matter how potent the medicine donated, the patient will eventually die. What is the worth of such food and medicine, except the use it is put to by the recipient - and the giver? The successful beggar provokes the conditions by which begging is no longer required: both giver and recipient are trained and strengthened in mind, body and heart, so they develop friendship and goodwill. Consequently, even the beggar who passively receives gifts or donations is also imperfectly practicing.

The fire sacrifice begins by asking, by begging. Yet the manner of the asking matters quite as much as the manner of the giving. Asking, if accomplished correctly, provides an opportunity for a disinterested stranger to give selflessly, and possibly to cease being disinterested. Receiving, if accomplished correctly, provides an opportunity as well: to understand the purpose of sacrifice. For what purpose did the numerous beings sacrifice themselves and die to become food for the giver? For what purpose was this food sacrificed and given to another? Merely to become excrement and urine? For what purpose is the recipient in requirement of the strength and health this food provides?

It is not difficult to observe there are many people in our community in need of health and strength, in need of food. Or medicine. Or other help. There are very many people in our community in need of food who cannot access our food banks, or our healthcare, or our various social services. There are very many people in our community in need of friendship. We should not lose sight of the importance of friendship; it is easy to forget when someone is hungry, or sick, that friendship is even more important - friendship is the whole of holy life.

Why then do we socially contemn those who resource to the food banks, who take advantage of our hospitals, who require our social services - when they have done nothing regrettable? Should a poor person feel shame for wanting a piece of candy as much as a solid meal? When a person begs for the benefit of their family, they are providing for their family - and dutifully, honorably discharging their obligations. Why do we feel contempt for the abjectly poor, the homeless? If we saw the homeless enjoying candy, would we think their ability to enjoy such a treat makes them unworthy of further gifts, of proper sustenance and support? Is the beggar who eats only bread and water more worthy than one who might enjoy a candy?

There is an uncanny antagonism against such beggars. Our City has invested in numerous signs to dissuade giving to beggars, suggesting that giving will not bring an end to their poverty. As if this is the reason a person should give to beggar - to end their poverty? There is antagonism against beggars, the expense and difficulty our City has gone through to prevent them from sleeping on public benches or other rest areas, in the public parks, or other places of resort is worth considering against the resistance we have in providing the homeless with proper places of resort, with adequate sanitation and police service. We regret giving them police service, and sanitation - we regret giving them subsidized healthcare, and food. We infringe upon their rights to vote, as if they were not our equal citizens.

There is nothing shameful in begging or poverty, even if these spiritual practices are undertaken involuntarily. Indeed, they are beneficial, whether undertaken voluntarily or involuntarily. Poverty is not a failure, or a weakness - or anything shameful. Not any more than wealth and strength is a source of pride or a sign of success.

That we have permitted our poor to become a public health hazard is without a doubt a fact. They fester in disease, and foment crime. Yet this is certainly our own fault - for they lack healthcare, sanitation and protection we are able to give. But perhaps there is some blame to bestow upon these beggars - for they have not succeeded in obtaining their needs.

A successful beggar must not permit themselves to become passive recipients of donations, nor may they permit themselves to lose sight of the duty and honor in their begging. A beggar must not permit their patrons from losing sight of the purpose and honor in giving. If we have become selfish and greedy, if we have lost our ability to perform such a small sacrifice, it is perhaps their fault. Indeed, when undertaken as a spiritual practice, beggars present an asset to the community we presently lack.

Reducing waste and recycling

Ananda instructed King Udena in the practice of recycling and reuse. When new robes were received, the old robes were reused as blankets, the old blankets reused mattresses, the old mattresses reused rugs. Eventually, old rugs wear out and must be recycled: cut into cleaning rags. Old rags were recycled by shredding them, and mixing the shreds with clay and used to repair buildings. (Vinaya II, 291).

Some things have changed since then: buildings today are of different construction and are not so easily repaired, to begin with. But the practice can be adapted by understanding the principles of reuse and recycling.

Reuse is the process by which an item, which had been acquired for one purpose and now no longer is suitable or sufficient for that purpose it was intended for, becomes useful to another purpose. Reuse is also known as "repurposing." Adapting the example above, an old blanket may become unsuitable for use as a blanket - becoming too dirty, worn or faded. But without modification, the blanket may be moved from the bed to the floor, and used as a rug. Or moved to the table for a table cloth.

Recycling is the process by which an acquisition is reduced to its elemental components, and then these elemental components are repurposed as the materials required for the construction or acquisition of a new item. Adapting the example above, an old shirt (few people wear robes out and about anymore) may become worn or unsuitable to its purpose of presenting a person as ready for work or business. However, by cutting that shirt into squares, that shirt has been reduced to elemental components of "cloth" and this cloth may be used to make rags. Or the cloth may be reduced further into elemental components of "threads" and utilized in the manufacture of kindling, stucco, plaster, etc. Notice, stucco and plaster are themselves elemental components required for the construction of other items. Similarly, an old blanket can be utilized as an elemental material of cloth to manufacture a pillow case - or a place mat.

Though Ananada extolled recycling and reuse, this is only one component of the training rule. Gotama also frequently instructed also in reducing consumption to what was necessary. Just as eating too much - or too little - can result in distress, disease and discomfort, acquisition must be undertaken in moderation as well. When something breaks, it is necessary to repair it - but only to a certain, moderate extent. While the actual extent depends upon the cost of repair vs the opportunity to save those costs by reuse or recycling, a good rule of thumb is to permit an item to be repaired five times before recycling or reusing it.

When is waste loss? Honoring Laxmi

It is undoubtedly a mistake and wrongdoing to waste things. But this cannot be avoided - and is in fact the necessary sacrifice to honor Laxmi.

The Arthashastra describes how, in any practice of manufacture, industry or commerce, there is always inefficiency and waste. The cost of minimizing the waste should not exceed the waste conserved: to spend time, effort and money saving something worth less than the resources invested in saving it is not wise.

There are also materials which naturally spoil and waste, or which must necessarily be wasted: for example, an orange prepared for eating has a peel which is not eaten, composts poorly, and has virtually no use at all. And some byproduct materials, like stone chips from carving a statue, have only low uses (if any use at all). While the peel might be manufactured into a spice, or in other ways utilized, there is a limit to how much spice is useful to produce. And the stone chips might be made into gravel, but the cost of saving that waste may exceed the value of the secondary production. Food eaten will result in waste which must be disposed of to avoid disease.

Waste is clearly seen in retail or service: these necessarily add a margin to the final product. These margins of brokerage are earned, and not wrong. As are the revenues earned by lending money. The cost of borrowing, the cost of purchasing from a broker - these are not wasted. Neither are the wastes of any other life function.

Mistakes can be costly, but the error is not wasted. It is a process of learning. Laxmi is a good teacher, but demands this fee: there is a cost to learning, whether from a tutor or from Laxmi directly (by experience).

Anything to be gained or prevented from loss, all Artha, must be worth the effort. And sometimes this means permitting loss. Just as it sometimes means not permitting loss. Understanding when to permit loss, and how much it may be diminished, is the result of practice.

Training in readiness

When you notice a person begging food, do you regret having no food to share? You should anticipate your regret, and bring food to share.

Did you humiliate them in the sharing, or honor them? Did you help the beggar accomplish their purpose? Did you accomplish your own?

When you notice a person begging food, and you have food to share, do you regret sharing? You should anticipate your regret, and defend what is not theirs to ask for.

The schoolhouse bully stealing lunch money, the luckless beggar, the relative in hunger, the poor stranger hungry after a long workshift, to whom do you have the first duty?

Is anything truly yours?

Bleeding yourself dry harms those who depend on you, for you have given their blood in your veins. Failing to give blood at all is a fault as well, for you have deprived those who depend on you the opportunity to benefit by their sacrifice of you.

There are so many complications to consider: readiness is not only carrying food to give, but knowing when and how to give it. Each experience, each moment of learning, every moment of practice, helps prepare you to perform.

Spring cleaning done right

It's time for spring cleaning, and many are taking advantage Grand Junction's generous trash service to throw out items they have been holding onto too long. However, it is easy to notice that many of these items are still usable, and could be donated to local non-profits - or gifted to even better benefit. And, much of the trash that remains is recyclable.

Spring cleaning is an excellent practice: it is not good to acquire and hold onto things unnecessarily, and each of us gains great personal benefit from letting go of those things we no longer need. However, there are better ways to discard our over-numerous possessions: it is possible to not only personally gain from the spring cleaning, but to permit others to advantage from our practice.

Selfishly depriving others of the use of our former possessions is easy, and sometimes comforting. Saying that what we give up "is useless, to me or anyone else. It is trash," makes the letting go easier. It is much more difficult to consider the needs of those strangers in our community that are impoverished, or even our impoverished relatives, and friends, are not so different than our own. It is very difficult to understand that the difference lies only in economic means to easily acquire what we need. And it is exceedingly difficult to respect our belongings sufficiently to understand the quality and beauty of their workmanship and utility has exceeded our own requirement, and these once-precious items are worth sharing with another who needs them. To understand these items seem cheap and affordable enough to us to presently discard, only because of our great economic strength.

Understanding our economic strength implies our responsibility – toward the empowerment of those who are weaker, and to the improvement of our community by leadership.

Perversion

There are four perversions, four wrong-views resulting from improper use of mind. First, a person may confuse what is constant with what is inconstant. Second, a person may confuse what is pleasant with what is painful. Third, a person may confuse what is self with what is not self. Fourth, a person may confuse what is desirable with what is undesirable. These perversions result in insanity, and restlessness, loss of satisfaction and the ability to become satisfied, an inability to become free from distress.

Stories of Dharma:
Vishnu, the player (actor, athlete)

Rasa Lila

It is easy to forget that the famous story of the Rasa Lila is as much about Kamadev as it is about Krishna and Radha.

It is the story of Kamadev's greatest battle. Kamadev, who was an avatar of Vishnu (quite as much as Krishna), had been invincible, and had even sought to attack Brahma. Upon his victory against Brahma, Kamadev recognized he was developing pride. Kamadev began to think that he was entirely invincible, or matchless. Understanding his danger from pride, he complained aloud that no one could defeat him, and he would be defeated by pride. Upon hearing his own complaint, Brahma said to Kamadev that he should visit Krishna on the full moon in the autumn: Krishna was a worthy adversary!

Increasingly, he was convinced he should test himself against Krishna: if, there, in the company of all the cowgirls he felt any love, he would know that he could be himself conquered. If not by the cowgirls, than by Krishna, himself - but if he still felt nothing, or caused Krishna to be overcome, then he would know that he must submit to pride - for doubtlessly then, he must be invincible. Even when pitted against himself. Kamadev was decided: he would battle Krishna and finally know if he was invincible, or matchless.

This is not the first time that Vishnu helped himself. Rama-With-The-Axe helps nearly every other avatar of Vishnu, and frequently, Vishnu's several avatars help each other.

Krishna, becoming aware of Kamadev's intentions, prepared for battle. Krishna armed himself with Maya, but was inexperienced in the Yoga of Maya: yet he could think of no other way to either defend himself, or overcome Kamadev. His strategy was to conquer Kamadev by making sufficient illusion to cause Kamadev to love him, Krishna: while Kamadev was anticipating Krishna to make him fall in love with the cowgirls, Kamadev would never anticipate that Krishna would become the subject of Kamadev's love! So Krishna, to the limit of his ability in the Yoga of Maya made it seem a perfect night for love: flowers bloomed, the full moon shown, a gentle, cool breeze blew from the banks of the river Yamuna. He then played an enchanting tune on his flute, and beautified himself. He danced there, in the moonlight among the flowers, in the evening breeze. He became quite beautiful, indeed!

Krishna's maya could not be ignored, and soon, all the cowgirls, all the women nearby, were attracted to Krishna, and came running the spot - the cowgirls and women, it must be remembered, are not merely cowgirls, but are embodiments of elements of the Dharma, are in fact elemental components of Vishnu. They are not avatars or manifestations of Vishnu, they are like limbs, or part of Vishnu, having taken the form of people to be near to Vishnu in his manifestation as Krishna.

The women crowded Krishna, and began to dance with him. Krishna's maya made them so beautiful! Krishna was concerned for their safety, this was no place for them: it was to be a battlefield between Krishna and Kamadev and already the cowgirls were being afflicted by maya! He encouraged them to go home to their families, to their husbands and children and cattle. "Do not be so easily enchanted, leave mundane lusts behind!" But the cowgirls refused to go, indeed they could not, for they were entranced, and trapped by Krishna's Maya. Every fiber of their being desired Krishna, and Krishna's victory. As Krishna worried for them, he began to care for them, and lost concentration on the Maya. And then he fell subject to his own Maya. He became entranced as well, and soon Krishna began to enjoy their company. This reciprocated love caused the cowgirls to develop selfish feelings, even individuality. This tore at the integrity of Vishnu, as he tore himself apart into numerous individuals. This tore apart the very existence of every world! As Vishnu began to shatter, and separate into individualities, Krishna teetered on the edge of destruction and defeat. And then he vanished!

To the cowgirls, who remained, and were still suffering from individuality, it seemed that Krishna was gone. They were distressed beyond words - not only at the defeat, but at the loss of Krishna to them (they were also still enchanted by the Maya), and their role in his defeat, when they so desired his victory. They refused to believe that Krishna was actually gone, for if he had been destroyed, they would have also. They were Vishnu as well! So they looked all over for Krishna, asking the plants and animals where he was hiding. Then they followed his footprints, and saw Radha's footprints beside him. The thought came to them that Krishna had carried Radha to some hidden place, for the purposes of enjoying her company better. It must be remembered here that Radha is none other than the avatar of Laxmi, Vishnu's wife.

Though Krishna and Kamadev thought they were battling each other only, in fact Radha had joined the fight to defend Krishna. Radha had noticed things going very wrong and suspected Kamadev, invisible somewhere, had also been using Maya, taking advantage of Krishna's relative inexperience in the Yoga of Maya. Radha acted immediately and saved Krishna from destruction.

Laxmi was a master of Maya, because she was Maya. So she chose as her weapon Maya, like Krishna and Kamadev. And at the moment before his defeat, she wove her own illusions and begged Krishna to carry her wherever he would wish, and do with her whatever he would wish. She enticed Krishna to leave the battlefield, that he might regather himself - both literally, by unifying his dividing individuality, but also in formulating a better strategy against Kamadev who would have won the day.

Krishna was utterly entranced by Radha. This was not only because she was a greater master of Maya than even Kamadev, but because of his love for Radha. Krishna-Radha merged in this love, and Vishnu was healed somewhat of his injuries. Vishnu, as Time, held the world still; Radha and Krishna danced in an endless night of joy, for years, hundreds of years, thousands of years, epochs of ages. Radha's love permeated all of Time, all of Vishnu. And the cowgirls, restored through Vishnu's health, danced and celebrated the love of Krishna-Radha with them; in Time, Krishna was healed.

Kamadev now cared nothing of secrecy and invisibility. Kamadev revealed himself, and fired arrow after arrow at Radha! Her illusion defeated, Radha revealed herself as Laxmi, and defended herself against every arrow; even while dancing with Vishnu, she was fighting Kamadev, Laxmi was inexhaustible. As Kamadev was about to be overwhelmed by Laxmi, Kamadev remembered his true fight was with Vishnu, and his purpose for the battle. He would not be destroyed without firing at least one more arrow at Krishna! Besides, there was only one who could overcome Laxmi, and that was Vishnu himself. He would confuse Vishnu, and make him fight against Laxmi! (Now Kamadev had also forgotten who he was - Vishnu, and that he might have defeated Laxmi. All three combatants were highly intoxicated by the Maya).

With this last arrow, Krishna was terribly injured; he turned against Laxmi! Krishna saw Radha had used Maya against him, and began to misunderstand that for aggression. Ensnared by Maya, Krishna was so confused. Was Radha his enemy too? No, his love was too real to be obscured by Maya. Krishna loved and trusted her; she was a part of him. So Krishna reasoned Radha believed herself superior to the other cowgirls, and sought to seduce him. Thus, Krishna separated from Radha, and reminded her of her original request. he lifted her onto his shoulder. He was going to teach Radha a lesson - lifting Radha up, he disappeared right under her, letting her fall to the ground. Krishna left the battlefield.

Radha cried out in pain and surprise, but was consoled that her plan had worked. Krishna was safe, for the moment, from Kamadev. She was quickly found by the other cowgirls. Radha explained the situation, and suggested they return to the banks of the river to help Krishna.

They began to cry out to Krishna, reminding him of who he really was by recalling all of Vishnu's names and deeds. They tried to remind Krishna of what was real; by the instruction of Radha, they dispersed all the illusion, all they Maya. Then, dismayed, they wept, thinking Vishnu would never be wholly healed. This stirred Krishna's compassion, and he finally woke from the illusion to understand what had happened. He gathered himself, and reappeared among them.

Krishna was now more beautiful than before; he was not even trying to be beautiful - he actually was more beautiful now. Krishna explained he had been trying to teach Kamadev a lesson, but his own pride blinded him to his inexperience with Maya Yoga. His inexperience made him not really understand beauty. So, when he tried to entice Kamadev, he ended up enticing only himself - the cowgirls - he nearly destroyed himself with Maya, for the cowgirls were a part of himself. In the grip of his own Maya, Krishna mistook his own pride for theirs, and tried to teach them a lesson by disappearing. He forgot they were part of him. As he forgot even Radha was a part of him. He and they each grew more separated by this. Radha had reminded him of what true beauty was, and then Krishna understood his own pride prevented him from mastering Maya. Their efforts to disperse the Maya reflected his own efforts internally to wake from the illusion and defeat his pride, for they were one and the same being.

Krishna, now able to understand, was instructed in Maya Yoga by Radha, and learned sobriety, learned to refrain from desire, from emotion - and thus, as a master of Maya, defeated Kamadev: Krishna had conquered himself, and taught himself a lesson - and this inspired the undying love of Kamadev, who was also one and the same as Krishna, quite as much as any of the cowgirls.

Vishnu had made himself worthy of his pride, and in doing so, conquered it.

Sitalsasthi - the birth of Kamadev

Shiva was so deeply grieved by the death of Sita that he forgot the basic nature of things, and who Sita really was. When Parvati again manifested Shakti, Shiva was so grieved by the loss of his Ardhangini that he did not notice his Ardhangini was again standing before him. After the death of Sita, Shiva undertook profound Sannyasa, and by Hatha misused renounced Kama. In renouncing Kama, he renounced all his work, his Artha.

In renouncing his work, he renounced his duty, his nature, his Dharma. And so Shiva slipped from meditation into sleep.

When Shiva renounced his work, terrible evil arose in the world. Tarak the Asura prosecuted the ancient war between the Asuras and the Devas with vicious success, having obtained a blessing from Brahma that he would only be killed by a son of Shiva. Tarakasura thought that since Shiva would bear no child except with his Ardhangani, and his Ardhangini was dead, and even if she was again manifested Shiva would not see her because of the delusion of his grief, that he would be safe forever.

When the Devas asked Vishnu for help against Tarakasura, Vishnu suggested that they awaken Shiva, and show him his Ardhangini was again by his side. But while most of the Devas could not wake Shiva, those who did failed to help Shiva see that Parvati had manifested Shakti, and was his Ardhangini. All the beings tried to wake Shiva, and show him - but none succeeded. Vishnu knew, though, that one of the Devas had not tried.

Kamadeva is an Avatar of Vishnu. Kamadeva had manifested Vishnu to become the most powerful being in any world. He was victorious against even Brahma, and had defeated Shiva before. But Shiva promised that the next time that Kamadeva attacked Shiva, Shiva would utterly destroy Kamadeva. Knowing the importance of Kama to Artha, and ultimately to Dharma, for the sake of the universe, Kamadeva stayed well away from Shiva.

Now, Kamadeva was the only one who could succeed, and was called upon for a suicide mission. Rationalizing that there would be no use for Kama without Dharma, and that Tarakasura was destroying the Dharma, the Devas persuaded Kamadeva to sacrifice himself. Kamadeva knew that he would be destroyed, so before he left on his mission, he said a goodbye to his wife, Rati. Rati was also his vehicle, and he did not want her also hurt in the battle with Shiva. Rati said she could not live without Kamadeva, for they were one and the same; Kamadeva said this would be the reason he could again return to her. As Sita returned to Shiva, he promised so would he return to Rati.

Kamadeva began his work by first transforming Parvati into Uma, an irresistible beauty. Instructing her to stand before Shiva, Kamadeva prepared himself for the moment of his ending. Kamadeva did not have to sneak up to Shiva, he was so deeply asleep. The instant that Kamadeva struck Shiva, he awoke, and saw Parvati, and loved her. Kamadeva, fully understanding his mission, inspired sexual desire in Shiva, and he instantly copulated with Parvati. Thus, Kartikeya was conceived (incidentally, so was Hanuman - but that is another story). Kartikeya would come to defeat Tarakasura.

Shiva was so very happy that his Ardhangini had returned - and pleased beyond joy by his sons. But when he understood that Kamadeva had attacked him, he remembered his promise with some regret. Kamadeva knelt before Shiva in surrender, but not defeat. To Shiva's surprise, Kamadeva encouraged Shiva to fulfill his promise to destroy him, and all his promises - but to be more careful in making promises in the future: for sometimes a friend is required to harm a friend, as Kamadeva had harmed Shiva to wake him. Sometimes, even lovers fight, and hurt each other. Even in the most intimate ways. Kamadeva professed his love for Shiva, his brother, and called upon his brother to fulfill his promise. Now, it was Shiva's turn to harm Kamadeva: Kamadeva was at the verge of being overcome by pride, and needed to be awakened too. Shiva, ever more grateful to his brother, Kamadeva, was unable to refuse Kamadeva and burnt the brave Kamadeva with his third eye. Shiva utterly incinerated Kamadeva.

There was nothing left of Kamadeva, and Rati grieved profoundly. But Shiva reminded her of what Kamadeva had said to her. Kamadeva would fulfill his promise. Rati was confused - how was this possible? And thus, by profound effort, she understood. She manifested by her love of Kamadeva the Avatar of Kamadeva - in the womb of Krishna's wife Rukmini, as Pradyumma. Vishnu, as Krishna, also missed Kamadeva, and had manifested the Avatar in the womb of Rukmini. Rukmini, too, missed Kamadeva, and manifested Kamadeva in her womb. Rukmini, the wife of

Krishna, was also the Avatar of Laxmi; Laxmi is in the same way Rati, the wife of Kamadeva.

But because Shiva had destroyed Kamadeva at Kamadeva's request, there remained some doubt for a long time whether this meant that Kamadeva was truly invincible. Was Krishna a more powerful manifestation of Vishnu than Kamadeva? Krisha had never nor would ever be destroyed. Thus, Kamadeva and Krishna eventually tested their strength against each other in battle, and in mutual victory, completed the Self-Sacrifice.

Bhagavata Purana - Samkhya Yoga

This is what Vishnu said to Kapila.

Do you want to be free of love and hatred, the slavery of the senses and their endless torment of desire, to be free of the feelings of "I" and "mine," of self and possessions that rule your life? Do you want to be free of attraction and revulsion - of all the oppressive emotions that tyrannize and terrorize you? Do you wish to see beyond the veil of ignorance you have drawn across your eyes? Do you want to be free of the endless procession of becoming and ending? Are you yet weary of this prison, of Samsara?

Many Yogas lead to this freedom. Samkhya Yoga has led to this freedom from ancient times. In ancient times, it was learned that it is the mind that causes bondage - and liberation. When the mind becomes attached to the objects off the senses, it becomes embroiled in Prakriti, in unmanifested potentiality: the anticipation of ending and becoming is the basis of the three Gunas, the chains that bind you and torment you. The three Gunas are Sattva (Brightness, orderliness), Rajas (Confusion, activity), and Tamas (Darkness, chaos). These three Gunas cannot be balanced, and sooner or later, one Guna comes to dominate, and you become entangled in concepts of this and not this. This forms the basis of all instinctual reactions of pleasure and pain. This makes you restless, peaceless, and emotional. You become bound in the world of Ahamkara, the self, by wrongly understanding something as not-self.

But should you instead turn your mind from the senses, and instead turn your mind inward, you will find Me, Purusha. Your mind will calm as all impurities fall away from it. There becomes nothing to avoid or seek. There is neither this nor not this. You will understand detachment, Sannyasi. Understand that even the Atman is "this," and Anatman is "not this." You will understand detachment makes its own bonds - and loose yourself from them. You can become free, even from Freedom.

This is the perfection of Bhakti Yoga: the power of realization. The mind by itself is neither good nor bad, turn it outward to desire the objects of the senses and it binds. Turn it inward and it unbinds. For there is nothing there to bind to. The illusion of the self, the Atman, is the key to your freedom. Turn your mind to Me, Narayana, and all your obstacles will be broken.

Yet it must be a gradual path: the company of satsang, though, will hasten your progress. And if you ask who these true Sadhus are, whom you satsang should be composed of, seek those full of compassion. The sufferings that plague other beings, both physical and mental, do not affect these true Sadhus. They are kinsmen to all other beings, they have no enemies. They are always calm, in the face of even the most severest trials. They are always courageous. They never waver from the path of Dharma, but perform their duty without hesitation. They are unattached to all things of the world, they are senseless. They are ornamented by their honor, their character. Being with such Sadhus whose only preoccupation and concern is with Me will remove your own attachments, for it is the nature of the mind to be influenced by its environment, and companions. This is the purpose and use of Satsang: produce the environment and company conducive to your success.

Hear My stories, cheer your heart! Discover true pleasure, that which makes you seek the nature and cause of joy. Understand joy, and you will understand the purpose of Bhakti Yoga and all devotion: it is conducive to your success.

Satsang leads to Rati, Pleasure, and Rati leads to Bhakti. Bhakti lights the darkness, and illuminates the path of freedom. If you seek freedom, seek Me, seek the source of your Self, illuminate the darkness and see the illusion. Seek the source of joy. You will naturally become detached from the world of samsara understanding your senses, and their purpose. Do not act on illusion, act on logic, and reason. Even in the midst of illusion, in the mists of Maya, even in your bondage, you will be free!

I am always with my Bhaktis, they see Me everywhere; their senses are filled with Me, understanding Me. And by such understanding they obtain Moksha, whether they wanted it or not. They have become deathless. Even My weapon, the Chakra, the Wheel of Time, the Wheel of Dharma, which grinds all things down, is powerless against these Bhaktis. To my devotees, I am all things. Thus they have no fear of anything. Great and small, gentle and terrible, all that is sensed, are Me.

I am Nirvanatman, the one Free of Freedom, my Bhaktis become Freedom itself. Beings perform their Duty, their Dharma, in diverse ways. And those who perform their Duty desire nothing more. To perform their Duty truly, they ignore illusion, and by logic and reason, and become free from all distress.

Bhagavad Gita II, 42-53: standing steady

The flood of experience suppresses a thirst for knowledge...

Krishna said, the unwise take pleasure in the flowery words of the Vedas, saying "there is nothing else but this," when even "this" says it is nothing. Having cut the flower to enjoy it, they will never taste the fruit. Consequently, they are unsatisfied, filled with desire: they are driven by reward as their goal. With reward as their goal, they think in terms of reward, and think of all things as reward - or punishment. They think that birth is the reward for one's actions, and do not understand birth is a kind of distress. Confusing disease and cure, they prescribe pleasure, and delude themselves in the narcotics of power - that they might know greater reward, and less punishment.

Know then that the Vedas only deal with the gunas. If you are beyond these, freed from the illusion of duality between good and evil, between right and wrong, between even pleasure and pain, you will never suffer thoughts like these. To such a Brahmana, to one who has gone beyond, the Vedas and all knowledge are as much use as a tank of water when and where there is a flood.

Like an ox who pulls the plow, you have no right to the products of your work. And frequently, there is failure in a crop, there is no right to the harvest - but the seed must still be planted, the plow pulled, the oxen worked. Do not let the fruit of your actions be your motivation, do not be motivated by reward. Remain steadfast in the yoke, in your effort, in Yoga: do not let yourself lapse into inaction. Abandon your attachments, sacrifice them and you will be balanced in success and failure. Such evenness of mind is the yoke you must bear. Therefore, give up thoughts of good and evil deeds, of right and wrong, of success or failure. Devote yourself only to the skill of your action. Go beyond. Beyond all wrong. Beyond birth. Free yourself from birth and evil.

If you will go beyond the Vedas (knowledge) you must fearlessly enter into the flood of experience. When you have crossed beyond the flood, then you will be indifferent to the Vedas. You will be indifferent to all the knowledge you possess, and all the knowledge you lack - as someone who has just crossed a flood has no desire for water. Having covered the extent of knowledge, you will become as indifferent to knowledge as you would be to a tank of water covered by a flood. Discover the limits of knowledge, find the other shore. Then you will stand steady, having understood.

Udana 2.1: the first enlightened lesson

Understandably, the first lesson Gotama gave to human students at the Deer Park is cherished, but the very first lesson Gotama gave upon his enlightenment was to Mucalinda, the Snake.

When Gotama just realized full enlightenment at Uruvela, beside the river Neranjara, he sat for a week recovering his strength, experiencing the bliss of freedom. Now, it happened that there came a great rainstorm out of season, with cold winds, and unsettled weather. With this came mosquitoes, gadflies, and all kinds of irritations. So Mucalinda the Snake, King of the Nagas left his palace and encircled Gotama's body with his coils and covered Gotama's head with his cobra hood to keep Gotama warm, sheltered from the rain, wind, mosquitoes, gadflies, and the other unsettled weather and irritants.

When the weather cleared, King Mucalinda removed his coils from Gotama's body and stood before the Buddha, in Bhakti Yoga. Gotama said to the King, "Detachment is blissful - if you are content, have learned the Dharma and see. Such bliss is actually non-affliction; expressed by restraint toward other beings and all irritants. One who overcomes desires for pleasure and aversion to pain is blissful, this is possible by abolishing the conceit of "I am.""

Dasaratha Jataka: the former life of the Buddha, as Rama

The Buddha Gotama said,

once upon a time at Benares, the good King Dasaratha had two sons and a daughter with his Queen-Consort: Rama, Lakkhana, and Sita (daughter by marriage to Rama). In time, the Queen-Consort died, and the King was crushed by sorrow. But, urged by his court, the King set another wife in her place as Queen-Consort. This wife was also dear to the King, and in time as Queen-Consort she gave birth to a son named Bharata. The King was so happy with the birth of Bharata, that he offered to the Queen-Consort anything she would want. She strategically told the King she would ask the gift at a later time. And, when Bharata was seven years old, and Rama was to be given the Kingdom, the Queen-Consort asked her gift: "give Bharata the Kingdom."

The King was greatly enraged at this, and snapping his fingers at her, called her terrible names, and ordered her out. "My other sons shine like blazing fires, will you kill them and ask this Kingdom for the son of yours?"

She fled in terror, but encouraged by some supporters, continued to remind the King of his promise to give her what she asked for, and insisted on this gift. This caused the King alarm: that she had support, and determination, she might find a way to murder her son's rivals. So he called his sons together, and his court, and explained the situation to everyone gathered. He told Rama, "I cannot keep you safe if you remain here. Go to a neighboring Kingdom, or to the forest, and in 12 years when I am dead and cremated, return and claim the throne." Everyone wept when Rama promised to do as the King commanded. But then Lakkhana said he would go with his brother, and Sita said too, "I too will go with my brothers," and the three left the palace before the King could object.

When the three siblings left, they were accompanied by a vast company of people, who would have followed them into exile. But these were sent back to wait for Rama to reclaim the throne. The three siblings wandered a while, until they came to the Himalaya. There, in a spot near running water, convenient to wild fruit, they built an ashram and lived in hermitage.

Lakkhana and Sita told Rama, you are like our father to us, and will be King: remain here in the ashram. We will serve you, bring you fruit, and feed you. There they lived for nine years, while King Dasartha slowly died from grief and misfortune. When the King was dead, the Queen-Consort commanded that the umbrella be raised over her son, Bharata. But the Lords would not permit it, saying that the rightful heir was away in the forest. To his mother's surprise, Bharata himself also agreed with the Lords: "I will fetch back Rama, and raise the umbrella over him!" Taking the royal umbrella with him, Bharata led the Lords and army to Rama's ashram at a time when Lakkhana and Sita were away in the forest gathering fruit. At the door of the ashram sat Rama, undismayed and at ease. Prince Bharata approached Rama, and greeting him, standing at one side, told him of all that had happened, and falling at his feet with all the Lords and army, wept. Rama neither sorrowed nor wept, for he had no more emotion at all. Rama therefore comforted his half-brother, and they waited together for Lakkhana and Sita to return.

Rama considered in the quiet that if Lakkhana and Sita were to return now, they would be greatly pained at hearing that their father is dead: they had not yet accomplished the sacrifice of emotion, as Rama had. "Their hearts will break. I will persuade them to go down into the water, and there find a gentle way of telling them what has happened, the cool water will comfort them." So, he had Bharata, the Lords and all the army hide, and when Lakkhana and Sita returned, he gently remonstrated them. "You have taken too long harvesting fruit. Let this be your penance: go into the pond, and stand there.

When they were in the water, he joined them, and said "Bharata says, King Dasaratha's life is at an end." Lakkhana and Sita fainted. But the water revived them. Again and again, they fainted and rose, and at last Bharata, the Lords and army could not stand idly by: they rescued them out of the water, and setting them on dry ground, wept all together. Yet all noticed that Rama did not weep, understanding this as a sign of his emotional control, his yogic accomplishment.

Bharata asked Rama for help, to teach all those gathered there how to overcome their grief. Rama said,

"When young, a child cries when they cannot keep a thing. But not only children do this: even those who are full grown will weep at loss."

Rama sang,

"Is this wise? The child, the old, the fool and the wise
The rich and the poor may be sure
Each one of us dies!
As sure as you are ripened fruit will fall
As sure as you know by the evening the morning will be gone
The fear of loss, and death, is known to all."

Rama said, "What good does weeping and tormenting one's self as a consequence of loss accomplish? Grief weakens you, makes you thin, and pale. This does not bring the dead to life, or return what is lost - but results in further loss, and more reasons to grieve. When a house burns, much is lost, sometimes death results. But a housefire is put out with water, not with tears."

Rama addressed everyone present, "I will protect and care for all my people, but cannot protect them from death. As I could not protect my father, the King from death. And he could not protect me. Yet to who remain alive I will be their King. This is how I may best explain the impermanence of things."

When Rama said this, all present understood impermanence, and gave up their grief. Promptly, Prince Bharata saluted Rama, and begged him to receive the Kingdom of Benares. Rama replied, "No, brother. My father commanded me to return after 12 years, and this I will do. Take Lakkhana and Sita with you, and administer the Kingdom yourselves until then." Bharata, Lakkhana and Sita objected, saying they could not: they lacked Rama's wisdom and ability. Rama assured them, though this might be true, they were nevertheless sufficiently competent. A Kingdom, well administered, did not even require a King. Taking off his sandals, Rama gave them to Bharata saying that even these sandals could administer the Kingdom - certainly Bharata, Lakkhana and Sita could do as well? With this, he said goodbye to his siblings, his Lords and army, and promised to see them again in three years.

For three years the sandals administered the Kingdom: when there was a case which required the King's judgement, the sandals were consulted. If the lower judge had decided a case incorrectly, the sandals were beat upon each other (by Bharata, Lakkhana and Sita), and the lower judge would re-examine it. If the decision of the lower judge was right, the sandals would remain quiet.

When the three years were over, Rama returned, came to Benares, and entered the park. When this was discovered, everyone came to the park to celebrate the return of their King! Sita was made Queen-Consort, and Rama and Sita were paraded clockwise around the city. Then, ascending to the palace Sucandaka, Rama reigned a long time, before death took him too.

The Buddha Gotama then concluded the story, saying in time, legends expanded the length of Rama's reign - so much did the people wish he had reigned longer. It became said that he reigned not for 60 years, but for 60 times 100, and then ten-thousand more (10,600 years). And if a pair of sandals could reign for three years, why not believe this? At that time, Suddhodana was King Dasaratha, Mahamaya was the mother of Rama, Rahula's mother (the Buddha Gotama's wife, Yasodhara) was Sita, Ananda was Bharata and I, myself, was Rama."

Agni Purana 1.3 – Boar Varaha

Vishnu was next manifested by the form of a boar. The sage Kashyapa and his wife Diti had a son named Hiranyaksha, who became the King of the Asuras. Hiranyaksha, by his righteousness, pleased Brahma so that Brahma granted him any wish: Hiranyaksha wished to be invincible in battle. Hiranyaksha thus went to war with the Devas, and because he was invincible in battle, utterly defeated the Devas and conquered the Devaloka. In the course of his war, he also conquered Varuna, the Ocean. Hiranyaksha was unstoppable! He became King of every world.

Of all his domains, Hiranyaksha enjoyed most of all the ocean, and came to live in Varuna's palace under the waters. But he also loved the Earth, and so he pulled Her down into the ocean to live with him, causing Her considerable misery.

By now, Brahma understood that, despite his good intentions, he had permitted something terrible to happen by granting this wish. So he led the Devas to Vishnu and asked that Vishnu do something about Hiranyaksha, and his despicable treatment of the Earth. The Devas should be restored to the Devaloka, and the Earth should be brought back from the ocean's depths. Vishnu agreed something should be done. But where was the Earth?

In the form of a boar, Vishnu entered the ocean - and frolicing and playing, swimming in the vast waters. This attracted the attention of the Earth, who fell in love with Vishnu; she called to him, and this is how Vishnu was able to find the Earth. He dived down, and lifted Her in his tusks, carrying Her out of the waters.

Hiranyaksha did not know that this boar was Vishnu, and thought it was an ordinary boar coming to steal his love. So he attacked the boar. Soon, it became apparent this was no ordinary boar! As they fought, Hiranyaksha saw the boar's feet were the vedas, his tusks were sacrificial stakes, his teeth offerings, his mouth an altar, his tongue the sacred flame! Too late, he understood: it was Vishnu, in the form of sacrifice itself! Vishnu bent time, and the battle stretched on for a thousand years. Vishnu wore down the will of Hiranyaksha, tiring him; the more Hiranyaksha fought with Vishnu, the more he admired Vishnu, and became reluctant to keep fighting. Hiranyaksha then at last understood he had done terrible wrong, and regretted that he had asked to be invincible: it was that gift that spurred him to try to conquer every world, and even fight Vishnu. Now, Hiranyaksha's pride was subdued, and he asked Brahma to take back the gift given him, and asked Vishnu to end his shame. Brahma agreed, and Vishnu gored Hiranyaksha with his tusks: the sacrifice restored Hiranyaksha's honor.

Upon seeing Her champion victorious, the Earth fainted, and began to sink under the ocean again. Once more, Vishnu lifted her up.

The Earth had fallen in love with Vishnu, and Vishnu recognized Her as his Consort; they married, and had a son, Naraka. But the Earth asked Vishnu for two gifts for their child: that he be all powerful, and have a long life. Despite the good intentions, these gifts ultimately led to Naraka becoming evil, like Hiranyaksha, and required both Vishnu (as Krishna) and the Earth (as Satyabhama) to subdue him, as well.

The Earth was so in love with Vishnu! But when at last Vishnu's play took him to a place hidden from the world, the world, like a woman bereft of her love, wondered how she might sustain herself against such unrequited love? The world sought the great Muni Kasyapa for guidance. The Muni suggested she seek her love, Vishnu, and lay bare her heart. The search brought the world far, but at last Vishnu was found: the world laid bare her heart to Vishnu.

Vishnu comforted her, he had never left: they were one and the same, inseparable, indistinct, she was her own lover. "Love those who practice their duties and act to uphold the Dharma as Me." With the world seated at ease in his company, Vishnu proclaimed many duties: to teach by sacrifice, to practice by protection, to care for and tender by commerce and industry, to serve through the arts. Forbearance, veracity, restraint, purity, liberality, self-control, harmlessness, obedience, pilgrimaging, compassion, straightforwardness, contentment, reverence, equanimity.

It is by action (karma) that we lift ourselves up. You rescued yourself.   It is by action we find what we search for. Have you found what you were looking for?

Kurma: turtle

Kurma Jayanti is the day Kurma, the nameless Turtle, manifested Vishnu. It happened during the churning of the oceans. On Kurma Jayanti, the nature of all those supernatural beings present at that moment can be reflected upon: they are merely other beings, and though very powerful, intelligent and beautiful, and worthy of respect, neither require nor deserve our worship - any more than someone who is less powerful, less intelligent, or less beautiful should be denied our respect. We are all (even those mighty devas) imperfect beings, in an imperfect world. We all share this world, and must work together as best we can, by helping out when we notice help is needed - as Kurma the turtle did.

Kurma was a giant turtle. Apart from his size, he was an ordinary turtle. At the time, all the beings were helping in the churning of the ocean of milk (the translation is poor, but "ocean" is used to convey the image of a vast amorphis mass which holds things dissolved within it, like the ocean holds salt, or "milk" holds fat in suspension). The nagas (snake people) gave their very bodies as ropes as the strong gods and demons pulled them back and forth to churn the ocean with the earth, which had given its mountains as the churning rod. Every being helped - to the extent they were able to.

Out of the churning came many wholesome and poisonous things. The poison threatened every world (in Hinduism, the multiverse is understood in terms of coexisting worlds intersecting each other at the same time, space or action). To protect the worlds, Shiva was manifested in all his avatars and vehicles, and swallowed the poison. In the same spirit, Kurma noticed the mountains slipping from the grasp of the snakes, and steadied the mountains - so that the mountains would not slip. This act of unhesitatingly providing help when needed at the moment it was noticed manifested Vishnu, and permitted the successful churning of the oceans.

But many good things came from the churning too.

The force of the churning, the "shakti," was none other than Laxmi (fortune and wealth) who was able to take form for the first time through the waves in the increasingly solid ocean. The first thing she saw upon taking form was Vishnu, and already in love with Vishnu, became his eternal consort: this is but a fancy way of saying that fortune and wealth are the manifestation of the force of cooperation, of living and working together in harmony: in Hinduism, stories are used as tools for understanding complex concepts symbolically.

Also out of the churning came the Apsaras (selfs, beings, spirits) - these were also able to take form, and helped with the churning. Varuni, a kind of wisdom, took form too, and began to argue and struggle with the Asuras - and has followed them around ever since (who hasn't struggled with their prior foolishness in regret upon gaining wisdom?). Numerous supernatural animals appeared, and fled this way and that. Among them came Kamadhenu, the condition of sacrifice (presented in the form of a lactating cow, who sacrifices her strength to nurture a calf). And there were several elephants, including Airavata. Indra wanted Airavata as his own vehicle, and left the churning to chase down and tame it. When the Uchhaishravas (a seven-headed horse) took form, it was caught by the Devas, and given as a gift to the Asuras as a sign of goodwill and friendship, and their patience with Indra as he chased down Airavata.

Numerous valuables emerged, including Kaustubha, the form of discerning valuation (which Vishnu was given, in honor of his love of Laxmi).

And the Parijat, a flowering tree that never fades or wilts, was presented in friendship to the Devas by the Asuras. Sharanga, the powerful bow, was a weapon that suited the belligerence of the Asuras. Chandra, the moon, became worn by Shiva.

But now Kurma Vishnu strained. In his strain, he broke apart. It was at this moment Dhanvantari manifested Vishnu: he was a physician whose medical skill Vishnu required - and now cared for Kurma, and all those who were weakening, sickening, and injured in the churning. At this moment, too, Shankha, Vishnu's conch, manifested when Vishnu could no longer pronounce "Om." This tool permitted the sound to be made, even though Vishnu was unable, manifesting the very last desire of Kurma Vishnu. And with it came music.

Laxmi, too, strained, and broke. She had begun to worry for Vishnu, and doubt his strength, and this worry and doubt manifested Jyestha, misfortune (an opposite of Laxmi's fortune).

The oceans grew warm from all the exertion, so Varuna pulled from the ocean an umbrella to shade the ocean from the heat of the sun. All beings united in the single desire that the churning would be finished, and this manifested the Kalpavriksha plant.

All the beings grew weary, and could barely move any more - as they fell from exhaustion, they manifested Nidra. And then, at the moment of utter exhaustion, Amrita took form from the ocean of milk! Amrita was success, immortality, victory - and was now to be stolen by the Asuras, who broke their promise to share with the Devas whatever emerged. They mustered what strength they had left and viciously attacked the Devas. But fortunately, Vishnu had anticipated this treachery, so no one got too hurt - and afterward Vishnu (manifested in female form as Mohini, irresistible persuasion and seduction) stole back the Amrita. So things worked out...but that is not part of Kurma's story, and is part of another story.

Yet the Devas, upon sharing in the Amrita, forgot to thank Vishnu for his help, though Vishnu had stolen back the Amrita, doctored all the beings who were exerting themselves, protected the Devas of the vicious attack and betrayal of the Asuras, and steadied the churning rod - nearly destroying himself in the process. Shiva was outraged on behalf of his brother's insult and approached the gods in the form of a yaksha (yakshas embody the nature of things or places or times or actions, almost like a soul or nymph). He complained that the Asuras gave better credit to Vishnu than the Devas did, because the Asuras at least blamed Vishnu for stealing back the Amrita - and then showed the Devas that as strong as they were, they could not have achieved success without every other being helping them. It is this lesson which is repeated by custom today.

Vaman: dwarf

The major manifestations of Vishnu are tied to a single family line through the ages. Hiranyaksha the Asura, who had been destroyed by Varaha the Boar who manifested Vishnu, had a brother, Hiranyakashipu, also an Asura, who swore vengeance on Vishnu. But Vishnu had no fight with Hiranyakashipu. Yet Vishnu destroyed Hiranyakashipu - he was destroyed by Narasimha, the half man half lion who manifested Vishnu, when he repeatedly threatened his son, Prahlada, and ignored Vishnu's warnings against harming Prahlada. Vishnu would destroy Prahlada's grandson as the Dwarf, Vaman, and Pralada's great-grandson as Krishna. The reason why Vishnu and the family of Hiranyaksha are so tied together is another story, but it suffices to explain that Vishnu had promised to instruct them in the means of destroying desire, hatred, and pride - "destruction" is not "killing," and is a catalyst for positive change and in this sense is akin to "sacrifice." Much as we would destroy or sacrifice a ruined old home to build a new one, or destroy or sacrifice plants in a controlled burn to contain a wildfire.

Important to this story, though, is that Prahlada the Asura was very good and righteous, and ruled honorably in his father's place. And Prahlada's son was an even better King than his father. And Prahlada's grandson, Mahabali, perfected the art of governance. It is said there was no criminality in the time of Mahabali, and every being was content with Mahabali's rule. This is interpreted two ways: first, in a literal sense: Mahabali perfectly upheld the Dharma. The second is sarcastic, suggesting the question of how there can be criminality in a state of lawlessness? The riddle is solved by understanding that law without mercy are unjust, that rules without exceptions are wrong: all laws and rules are, as the Buddha Gotama described them, "counterfeit Dharma." As Vishnu instructed as Krishna and the Buddha Gotama, the world needs criminal Dharma. It is senseless pride to believe that any rule or law can be perfected. A state where laws are fulfilled without mercy, and without exception, is as much a lawless state as any anarchy.

Mahabali sought to finish the war of the Asuras and Devas by conquering the Devas - and all the lokas, all the worlds. And he did. And then ruled them in his "perfect" governance. Law was upheld without exception, and there were soon no criminals. To recognize his triumph over criminality, and over every world, Mahabali announced a sacrifice in honor of Vishnu: he would give to anyone who asked him anything that they asked for. Vishnu saw this as a teachable moment about pride.

A dwarf, Vaman (for that is what "Vaman" means, "dwarf"), heard the announced sacrifice and, inspired by the profundity of the moment, manifested Vishnu. The dwarf was not only deformed by his condition, but also a cripple, having been horribly injured early in life, as punishment - representing the injury that Mahabali had done to the Dharma by his strict enforcement - much as a parent who injures their child in punishment has performed their instruction wrongly, and with catastrophic results.

The Dwarf brought himself by small steps to the throne of Mahabali, who, despite the instructions of Vishnu against sympathy (favoring instead compassion) felt sympathy for the Dwarf. Mahabali offered the Dwarf fine clothes and vehicles - these were declined. Mahabali offered the Dwarf gold and jewels - these were declined. All kinds of wealth Mahabali offered the Dwarf - livestock, food, comforts - all of which were declined. At last, Mahabali offers the Dwarf a measure of equality, some of Mahabali's Kingdom. This was a gift that the Dwarf could not refuse! The Dwarf gratefully accepted, but when Mahabali asked the Dwarf how much of the Kingdom the Dwarf wanted, the Dwarf said "not much. One must live within one's means. But a great King like you understands that! Perhaps you might give me all that might be contained within three of my small steps?" This the King agreed to. "Certainly I have conquered enough to share with you as much as you ask!" said Mahabali.

The Dwarf took one step forward, heart filled with Vishnu - and as he strode, suddenly he was healed, and grew in stature: growing to be the size of a giant, his step encompassed the entire world! The former Dwarf then took another step and grew in stature even more: this step encompassed every world! Where would he step next? Mahabali recognized the manifestation of Vishnu and said, "Vishnu, you have nowhere else to step, and I promised you three steps: in my pride, I thought I had enough to satisfy you. All that I have conquered is insufficient, all my righteousness is pretentious. You have humbled me. Stand upon my head, and claim all that is within my being? This last I do not reserve from you, and indeed it is all that I ever had to give." The offer was genuine, and kind, an act of supreme devotion. Vishnu, to fulfill the promise made generations ago, then stepped on Mahabali's head - but since Mahabali had destroyed his own pride, there was nothing to destroy.

Mahabali was liberated from his pride, and in his freedom was grateful to Vishnu. Vishnu was so proud of Mahabali - he had learned the lesson of humility himself! He had not needed to "break" or "destroy" Mahabali. All of Mahabali's subjects saw the moment of Mahabali's victory over pride, and were so proud of Mahabali, too! They desired him as their King forever and ever.

But Mahabali now did not want to rule, and claimed the right of renunciation, and renouncing all the worlds and his Kingdom, to devote himself wholly to Vishnu as a Sannyasi. Yet Vishnu persuaded Mahabali to return to the worlds once every year: he had a duty to his subjects, after all!

So Mahabali does return once every year, on Onam, and give gifts to anyone who desires anything, and gives true justice to those who require it - mercy where it is required, and strict enforcement where it is required. And, of course, to teach the value of humility.

Narasimha: lion

In the Vishnu Purana 1.11 - 1.14, and elsewhere, the story is told of Hiranyakashipu, who received a gift from Brahma after devoted yogic study, practice and service. The gift he requested was eternal life, but Brahma said that because even Brahma would not live forever, this could not be given. So, instead, Hiranyakashipu asked that he will not be killed either by a man or a beast nor any kind of being at all, neither will he be killed indoors or outdoors and nor during day or night, not in his home or away from his home, not by any weapon, not on the ground nor in the ocean, and not in any way that his dead body (or even a drop of his blood) would fall to the ground. This Brahma willingly gave.

What Hiranyakashipu then did was go to war against his enemies, the gods. Because of Brahma's gift, none of the gods could stop him - he conquered the devaloka, and enslaved the gods: even Surya, Vayu, Agni, Varun, Chandrama, Kuber - even Yama was overcome. With the gods overthrown, Hiranyakashipu quickly conquered every other world. But what he did not understand, despite his studies, was that Vishnu was not a god and he thought that Vishnu was a god, and his enemy. He commanded that Vishnu no longer be worshiped.

But his eldest son, Prahlad, though only a child did understand better. He tried to explain to his father that Vishnu was not his enemy. He said to his father this, and his father summoned all the child's teachers - demanding who had disobeyed him to teach Prahlad Vishnu was not his enemy. All the teachers denied teaching him this, and the boy vouched for them - he explained that he had figured out for himself that Vishnu was not his enemy.

The boy said, Vishnu is beyond form, beyond existence, and is therefore in every heart. Even within his own, and his father's. This greatly upset Hiranyakashipu. But his son continued to insist, Vishnu was everywhere, and at all times. His father grew angry, and asked if Vishnu was the king of every world? The boy explained, that since his father was the king of every world, so was Vishnu. His father was utterly confused, "you're babbling!" he told his son.

But Prahlad continued to insist that Vishnu was everywhere, and at all times. His father commanded him to stop saying this. "But it's true!" complained the child. Hiranyakashipu commanded that anyone who said this would be put to death, and told the boy's teachers to make sure that when the boy returned before him again that he knew better. Months passed. But the boy refused to accept what his teachers told him, for he understood that Vishnu was not his enemy, and was everywhere and at all times. At last, Hiranyakashipu called his son before him again, and asked him what he knew about Vishnu. The boy said, "though whoever says so will be put to death, it is nevertheless true that Vishnu is not our enemy, and is everywhere at all times."

"I shall prove to you that Vishnu is not everywhere and at all times, and is not your friend," said Hiranyakashipu. He ordered his bodyguards to attack the child. But the child merely said, "Vishnu is in me, and in your swords, and in you. I will not be hurt by Vishnu because Vishnu is not my enemy." The child expertly dodged every blow aimed at him. Eventually, the bodyguards had to give up. Hiranyakashipu praised the martial skill of his boy, "you have learned your lessons well, and ably dodge weapons! I would pardon your life, if you will only stop praising my enemy." But the boy remained determined, "I am not praising your enemy: Vishnu is not your enemy. And in understanding Vishnu is everywhere and at all times, I have no fear of death."

Hiranyakashipu then had his son thrown into a pit of poisonous snakes. But as he was brought to the edge, the boy said, "Vishnu is in me and in the snakes, I will not be hurt by Vishnu because Vishnu is not my enemy." And, laying still among the snakes, utterly without fear, he was not bit. Hiranyakashipu had his son taken out of the pit. "You are very courageous! I would pardon your life, if you will only stop praising my enemy." Again, the boy defied his father. But now, there were whispers heard that the boy was superior to his father in courage and martial skill -

would his father have conquered every world if it had not been for the gift of Brahma?

Now Hiranyakashipu feared his son as a threat to his throne. To demonstrate his dominance, he caused elephants to stampede toward the boy - but the boy remained still, and was not harmed - for he understood Vishnu was in the elephants, and Vishnu was not his enemy. "You may have the gift of Brahma, but I have knowledge of Vishnu," he told his father. "Vishnu is not your enemy. And neither am I." Now, the boy's teachers begged Hiranyakashipu to stop trying to kill his son, to give them one more chance to re-educate the child. This mercy was granted, and the boy was saved - until the next time he was called before his father, the King.

But at the school, Prahlad began to teach his teachers. " Every living being is born, suffers during life, and dies. Yet every being easily mistakes hunger, thirst, cold, and heat for pleasure and pain. The more luxury one collects, the more one's sorrow increases. Attachment and desire are the cause for sorrow. And even after all this sorrow, after the agony of life and death, there is no end to the distress - like an ocean which one cannot drown by, but sinks deeper and deeper into. But sure as all that is born must die, all that ends must begin again."

Prahlad said to his fellow students at the school, "Do not be confused by my youth. I may have the form of a boy, but I have eternally existed. There is no time, no place, no growth, no becoming, no ending for Me. Yet in taking such form, there is a lot of misconceptions - a boy would rather play than be contemplative. In youth, lust and carnal pleasure attract his mind. Spiritual matters are postponed until old age - but then, the mind and body are already weak - and gained nothing by his play and pleasure. The wise person realizes that this form is transitory, and understand what he has to do now. Understand right now that Vishnu is everywhere, and at all times - and you may understand your duty also exists beyond time and space." The children were convinced, and soon taught their teachers, too.

News of this came to Hiranyakashipu, who ordered his cook to poison Prahlad. But Prahlad, for some reason or another, did not die. This frightened the cook, who then became a student of Prahlad.

The teachers were then ordered to kill Prahlad. But they decided to try to save Prahlad one more time. "It is not good to be disobedient to your father, or to violate the law." But when Prahlad explained that Vishnu was not his father's enemy, it was neither crime nor disobedient to praise Vishnu. And a child has a duty to protect his father from making an enemy unnecessarily, to insist upon the truth - this truth had been proven many times now. Some of the teachers fled, rather than kill the boy, disappearing beyond the worlds. Those who remained saw his father's command through: they ordered the executioner, Kritya, to kill the boy. She struck the boy with her trident, but it shattered, and the fragments killed those teachers who had ordered the execution.

Prahlad was very sad at having none of his teachers. Speaking to Vishnu, he asked that they all be brought back to him from death, from beyond the worlds. Vishnu restored all of Prahlad's teachers, and encouraged them to instead direct their efforts at re-educating Hiranyakashipu.

Hiranyakashipu began to suspect his son had developed magical powers - and refused to believe his proofs that Vishnu was not his enemy. He had his son thrown from a roof, he had his magician try to kill Prahlad - only to see the Sudarshan Chakra, the weapon of Vishnu, defend Prahlad. In desperation, Hiranyakashipu ordered the gods to try to kill Prahlad. But none of the gods could - even Vayu (wind) could not dry him. Once more, the teachers prevailed upon Hiranyakashipu to forgive his son, if only temporarily - maybe after he finished his education, he would understand things better?

Years passed. Prahlad did finish his education, and was called before his father. "Son, tell me what you learned about diplomacy." Prahlad said, "My teachers have taught me in many different subjects, including diplomacy - I have learned them all with heart. I learned that diplomatic policies should be applied to train friendship. But, excuse me, father, but as I see no difference between friend or enemy, it is my opinion these lessons were irrelevant. What is the use, when Vishnu is everywhere, and at all times? In you, in me, and all beings. Instead of seeking personal gain out of diplomacy, one should instead seek the benefit of all. It is by making our environment and those we share it with stronger that we are strengthened. Everyone longs for a throne and a big kingdom - but such power can only be retained through justice. There is no defense for the unjust, for those who do not perform their duty, and make an enemy of Vishnu."

Hiranyakashipu then kicked Prahlad and ordered him tied and thrown into the ocean from the devaloka. But when Prahlad was thrown into the sea from the devaloka, he displaced so much water with his impact that his binds broke and he stood on dry land, and was able to rush to the mountains to escape the returning water. Hiranyakashipu ordered things thrown in the path of Prahlad, to try to trip him, so he couldn't escape. But, of course, these piled up and Prahlad climbed on top of them to escape the returning water.

Vishnu appeared at the top, and said "Prahlad! I am so pleased with you, and your devotion. Ask any gift." Prahlad did not have to think twice, "May I always be a servant to your duty, may I always be so devoted to you, may I always remember you in my heart." Vishnu said he could not give this, because Prahlad already would always be his servant, and always devoted to him, and always remember him. "Ask anything else." Prahlad thought, and said, "may my father learn better wisdom." Vishnu said, "Prahlad, you already know he will learn better, in Time. Ask something else." Prahlad then thought harder. "But I don't want anything else!" said Prahlad. "I'd have to ask you now to suggest what I should ask for!"

In time, Hiranyakashipu decided to kill Prahlad himself. At dusk, he tied Prahlad to a pillar at the gate of his palace, and shouted abusively for Vishnu to prove Prahlad right. Where was Vishnu? His sword would strike Prahlad, not Vishnu - but he wished it would strike Vishnu! He swung his sword at Prahlad's head, but Prahlad ducked - and the sword struck the pillar. The pillar cracked and broke with the force - and began to appear like Vishnu - it became Vishnu, in the Narasima manifestation! Half human, half lion!

Narasimha grabbed hold of Hiranyakashipu's sword. Then Narasimha grabbed hold of Hiranyakashipu. Right then, at dusk (not day or night), at the gates of his home (not inside or out, not at home or away), Narasimha (not man nor beast nor any kind of being at all) lifted Hiranyakashipu off the ground (not on the ground nor in the ocean), and squatting, laying him across his knees, tore him with his sharp claws (not a weapon) and devoured him (not even one drop of blood fell to the ground). Vishnu, being everywhere at all times, in every form, cannot be stopped.

Prahlad ascended to the throne, and ruled justly.

But Narasimha, having eaten someone so hateful and fearful, became fearful and hateful himself. You could say, his meal had *disagreed* with him. He began to rage and threatened to destroy all the worlds. No one could calm him down - or even get near to him! Laxmi said to Shiva, if she could only get near him, she might calm him down. Shiva then assumed the form of a half-lion half-bird, and carried Narasimha high into the sky. Then he dropped Narasima - not to kill him (nothing could), but the fall did scare Narasimha so much that he passed out. Laxmi rushed to Narasimha, and when Narasimha woke, he recognized his love, his wife. She sang gently to Vishnu, and kept him calm while Shiva tore off the lion's skin, and the form of Narasimha, freeing Vishnu from the fear and hate. In gratitude, Vishnu gave to Shiva the skin, which Shiva now uses as a blanket to sit on - or for some warmth against the cold.

The Atharva Veda, 15.11

When you come to a house of a Vratya, a vow-taker, ask them: how was your night? Here, Vratya, is water: refresh yourself! Let things be as you wish, let things be as would please you, may you accomplish all your desires! When you come to the house of a Vratya, and they ask how your night was, the Vratya gains rest; when they offer you water, they satisfy their thirst; when they extend to you their good will, they become beloved, contented, and desireless, having accomplished all their desires. Help the Vrayta attain their desire if you would attain your own.

Rig Veda 1.174

Water gives food, food gives strength, strength gives victory. Your rain, Indra, protects us against hunger, want and defeat! Rain falls with and upon your victory, because of your strength - the rain falls upon our fields, swelling our rivers - without destroying our cities or fortresses. Your water guards the sacrificial fire from escape, becoming wildfire, permitting us to enjoy its light and heat within our fields and homes without fear of everything burning. Maghavan, you are the giver of Heroes, giver of wealth, the giver of victory when you give us food. You protect and preserve us, and save us when you achieve your own victory! Your victory is our own.

Week 11

SUMMARY.

Beginner's Class: Mastering yatra: endurance training. Addiction. Outdoor practice: finding the temples of Kamadev. Intermediate Class: Buddhism. Guided practice

Training methods

- Introduction to yatra havinq already been made indirectly in previous sections, mastery of yatra will be practiced until the student is ready for performance through endurance training, and especially outdoor practice.
- Guided discovery of one of the shrines of Kamadev.

Mastering yatra: endurance training

Endurance training is a practice that is beneficial to mastering yatra sufficiently to undertake its performance. Journeys can be long, tiring, and challenging. It is therefore appropriate to train in the four jnanas, especially in body and mind, to strengthen sufficiently to perform the duties required.

In theory, everyone will carry their own pack, and themselves the entire way: but this is seldom the case. There will be those who are stronger, or more practiced, or more fortunate in avoiding injury - and those who are weaker, less practiced, or more unfortunate. One of the best ways to train is to carry another's load, or carrying another entirely.

One of the greater dangers in carrying another's load, or another, is contempt. If someone is wealthy, or strong, or healthy, they do not deserve your envy. No one deserves or requires being bowed down to. Why then would the strong hold the weak in contempt? The weak do not hinder justice, hinder administration, hinder the performance of yatra (or any other Dharma). They are the reason for it.

Housekeeping, and other Parvati Puja, is an excellent practice. Waking early (or going to rest/bed late) to care for another, whether a spouse, a friend, or any other, to permit them the ability to recover their strength, to permit them to perform their own duties, to accomplish the work for which they are most suited, in acknowledgement of your friendship as a gesture of love and respect, or for any other loving reason, trains body and mind, and especially patience.

Athletic exertion in uncontrolled environments is also excellent practice. Hatha in the heat, hatha in the cold, early, late, thirsty, hungry, bright, dark - enduring discomfort permits performance under a variety of non-optimal conditions, permitting optimization of these non-optimal conditions. When the heat and cold do not bother you, you are better able to enjoy and delight in the performance when it is hot or cold. Challenge yourself: stare at a candle, see in the dark, exhaust yourself, find the limits of your strength and grow stronger.

Challenge yourself to understand more, every science, every art, every mathematical skill, every kind of work, in every kind of society, every kind of religion and practice, emulate and study, perform.

Practice surrounded by beauty and pleasure - and train yourself to not be overcome by beautiful or pleasurable things.

Master all your instincts by familiarizing yourself with them. Know the hopes and fears of barbaric life if you would prepare yourself to properly regard the false-comforts of civilization.

There is no limit to the advice which is practical or useful. Avoid habit, be flexible. Sleep on a hard mat or on the floor, eat nutritious foods, be healthy. And endure sickness. And age. And dying. Prepare yourself for every journey you will inevitably take.

Ending thirst

Many people, upon discovering they are addicted to something or another, will try to purify themselves by purifying their home. They will pour out all the alcohol in their house, they will flush the drugs down the toilet, they will throw away all their cigarettes, get rid of their marijuana, destroy their television, or in other ways attempt to purify themselves by purifying their home.

However, they mistake home for self. Purification of home does not result in purification of self. Liquor, once poured out, can be replaced, brought back into the house by the drunkard. Drugs, flushed down the toilet, can be replaced, brought back into the house. The smoker will get new cigarettes.

When the drunkard has conquered their thirst, their home will remain free of alcohol. Such victory occurs only after difficulty.

So it is the same with all great victories.

Excerpts from the Kamasutras:
Shrines of Kamadev

A person enters into the Ashramas of Sannyasa, Grihastha and Vanaprastha by acquisition. A Sannyasi has acquired a wealth of knowledge; but householders in the Ashramas of Grihastha and Vanaprastha have acquired material wealth by gift, loan, inheritance, gift, or by right of conquest. Having thus accomplished acquisition, they should take a residence in a community, city, village or otherwise in the vicinity of good friends, where their practice may continue to develop. While other duties of Dharma and Artha must be observed, these are the duties of Kama:

The home itself is a Temple. It should therefore be situated near clean water, and the home prepared for various purposes: it is a tool intended for use. It should contain at least two divisions: an outer and an inner one. Like the householder, it should be divided into at least two compartments or divisions: the inner space should be private; the outer space should be welcoming to visitors. It should be surrounded by a garden.

The outer space should contain a place to sit, and should be agreeable to see. It should be more than agreeable, it should be pleasing: there should be flowers, and perfumes to make it smell pleasant. There should be comforts for a guest, there should be a space on which refreshments may be laid. There should be a container for garbage and waste. There should be ornaments and decorations. There should be musical instruments, or a board for drawing, games to play, some dice, some books - or other entertainments. Outside the outer room, there should be pleasant birds, a place for spinning or carving or undertaking other diversions. In the garden there should be a swing, and pleasant places for sitting.

In the morning, the householder should practice hygiene: they should brush their teeth, apply limited quantities of ointments and perfumes to their body, ornament their body and examine themselves in the mirror - as they would examine their own behavior and self-control through insight. Bathing should be undertaken daily. Shaving, if done, should be undertaken in moderation - every five to ten days is sufficient. Sweat and soiled clothes should be promptly removed.

In Grihastha and Vanaprastha, meals should be taken three times every day; in Sannyasa, one or two meals suffice. At the breakfast hour wild animals should be cared for, and taught language; sporting diversions should be undertaken. A midday sleep may be undertaken, and after this, community, conversation and association with friends should be undertaken. At the dinner hour there should be singing and other entertainment, but the evening should be spent with only with the spouse, and family. Bedtime should be spent in agreeable conversation.

Occasionally, the daily routine of Kama duties is replaced by full-day activities and duties - such as festivals, social gatherings, parties, picnics, and the like.

At least once every year, people should gather in honor of Saraswati - by competitive skills. The best should be given rewards. Though many skills may be tested, it is appropriate to especially test in singing and other performance arts. After the competition, let the audience choose who should perform again - and let the audience act as an assembly, and perform in concert. It is the duty to hold this competition in lean times as well as prosperous times, as much as it is the duty of everyone to show hospitality to strangers. Even strangers should be welcomed to such assemblies and festivals.

In Kama Yoga, a satsang is accomplished when people of similar age, disposition and talents, who are fond of the same pleasures and loves, with similar degrees of education, sit together in company, engaging in agreeable conversation. The subject of discourse are to be pleasant ones, word games and tests of knowledge, performance of the arts of Kama. Compliment those who have adorned themselves best, who are the best in every art of Kama.

At such a gathering, sometimes beverages are served - some of which are bitter, others sour, some sweet. Some of which may be alcoholic. But intoxication - from liquor, or any other pleasure, should be avoided.

Sometimes, the gathering is held at a park, or in a picnic. The journey to the picnic is as important as the picnic itself. All the Dharmic, Arthaic and Kamaic duties of the day are performed in the park. Return home in the afternoon, bringing flowers and other treasures as offerings.

If the gathering is to be held near water, ensure that all dangerous animals have been taken out of the water, and that the bathing area is secured on all sides.

These are other social gatherings: spending nights playing games, going out on moonlit nights, celebrating the spring, picking wild fruit, eating delicious foods, and undertaking the sports and pleasures which are traditional or unique to a particular place.

All the above gatherings may be sufficiently undertaken not only in social settings, but by the sole company of spouses, or a family with children.

The only ones not welcome to social gatherings are the "parasite" - a person incapable of enjoying pleasure. And the "buffoon," the one who loves pleasure too much.

The ritual picnic is undertaken upon the festival of new leaves in the spring. But the practice is also undertaken periodically throughout the year, as required: the picnic is an act of profound Yoga, and represents a sacrifice to Kamadeva.

The devotee of Kamadeva knows the locations of the sacred shrines, and how to discover new shrines as well: they are too numerous to recount here.

In the morning after accomplishing the particular duties of their household, they shall go to the gardens, or parks, or forests and wildernesses, dressed beautifully and appropriately for the sacred occasion. The journey (Yatra) is itself an act of Tirtha, pilgrimage, and shall be undertaken with as much celebration and pomp as possible: songs, laughter, storytelling, bright colors - each caste, family and profession knows the special skills and traditions required of them at this occasion. The practices of Kirtan Yoga and Sankirtan Yoga should not be neglected.

Having arrived at the shrine of Kamadeva, the men and women will perform their usual secular daily duties - but in service of Kamadeva. Each caste and profession knows their special skills, and the proper devotions required by Kamadeva: this "secret" knowledge can either be transmitted by Teachers, Parents or others who would initiate a new devotee - or easily discovered through an observation of the other beings devoted to Kamadeva, or by profound Bhakti Yoga. A shrine is typically busy with numerous devotees, representing the many beings, each practicing with a single heart the same acts of devotion.

If the shrine has a place of water at the time of the pincic (some waters are seasonal), a ritual bath will be performed to refresh the pilgrims from their journey: sometimes only the feet are washed, sometimes the entire body is immersed: the specific rituals required of each shrine, and the practices of each devotee differ somewhat. However, prior to the bath, all dangerous beings shall be drive away from the water: all the poisonous animals and plants, all the spiritual beings who would cause harm to the devotees. Not only at the waters, but on the Pilgrimage journey, and at the Shrine. The benevolent beings should be admired, and welcomed - not only at the waters, but along the Pilgrimage journey, and at the Shrine.

Apart from dangerous beings, the only humans not welcome by Kamadeva's Shrines are the "parasite" - a person incapable of enjoying pleasure, but who would sap the pleasure of others. And the "buffoon," the one who loves pleasure too much.

The humans who are to be especially welcomed at the Shrine are the "Comedian," "Tourguide" and "Master of Ceremonies (MC)" are also welcomed, they can bring laughter, joy, contentment and happiness to any occasion: like Priests at the Temple, they ensure the devotion is performed perfectly. Also welcomed is the "Celebrity," the one favored by fortune and honor, whose very presence brings luck and honor. Also welcomed is the "Professor" - the one who is skilled in body, mind and heart, and who may help everyone perform their devotions of Kamadeva in the manner of a priest

Once the duties of the day are performed, there shall be undertaken by adult men and women an act of sacred courtship: there shall be held agreeable diversions: just as the quails or rams would fight to win the hearts of their beloveds, each man and woman shall demonstrate the sacred skills instructed by Kamadeva - to the extent that they have perfected these skills, and with the intent of winning and keeping the love of their beloveds. In particular it is an auspicious occasion for gaming, dice and cards, sporting, storytelling, joking, magic, fighting and demonstrations of the physical, mental and spiritual abilities, of proving strength, knowledge, and compassion, of proving faith in beauty, love and affection, of renewing and building bonds of friendship and family through loyalty. They shall instruct the children in the secret knowledge of the duties, devotions, traditions and rituals which will be required of them when they mature.

For the youth, this is the time for play, and spectacles designed to win and keep the friendship and family they share, to explore and discover the secrets of the shrine, to develop a sincere and profound love for Kamadeva, to explore the full potential of their adulthood and study and learn the duties, devotions, traditions and rituals of the picnic. Upon maturity and forming their own family, they shall in combining the duties, devotions, traditions and rituals of their two lineages develop a new combination, which shall be instructed to their children.

When the season is appropriate, the devotees should enjoy the sweet treats of wild plants: the young shoots, and fruits; the sweet grains and roots and sprouts. It is appropriate to decorate each other in flowers and beautiful plants. It is appropriate, too, to use the flowers and plants for mock-fighting, as darts, goads, wands, spears, swords, or other weapons. This is the time devotions should be made to the plants.

In the afternoon, prior to returning home, the devotees shall gather flowers or other trophies and treasures, that they may better practice Bhakti Yoga in devotion of Kamadeva at home.

As on ordinary occasions, an afternoon nap is permitted only in the summer months when the night is short, or for the elderly and ill.

Sometimes, the festival of the picnic continues overnight, or requires multiple days of Pilgrimage to arrive at the Shrine - if the moon permits light, devotees should go about in the moonlight, and perform those special rituals that require darkness: the moonlit walk, the stargazing, the fire rituals, the storytelling, etc. etc.

Sobriety and modesty should be practiced during the entire picnic to heighten the devotee's awareness of Kamadeva.

It is important to learn the particular customs of the district where the shrine resides, and to ensure that the customs of the district are practiced at the shrine - even if these customs are not your own.

The heart

This the Buddha said, "the Bodhisattva Avalokitesvara closely studied how he knew the truth of all things, he perceived that all five senses are empty. This is how he overcame his suffering.

"Avalokitesvara said, 'Form does not differ from the void and the void does not differ from form. Form is void and void is form. The same is true for my feelings, my perceptions, imagination and consciousness. I understand delusion, the characteristics of the void. I have seen all Dharmas are non-arising, non-ceasing, non-defiled, non-pure, non-increasing, non-decreasing. I have understood in the void there are no forms, no feelings, perceptions, imagination or consciousness. There is no eye, no ear, no nose, no tongue, no body or mind, there is no form, no sound, no smell, no taste, no touch or even imagination. There is no realm the eye can see until we come to the non-realm of consciousness. There is no ignorance, also no ending of ignorance until we come to the end of old age and the end of death. Until we come to eternal old age and eternal death. There is no truth in suffering – truly we do not suffer! Because there is no beginning of suffering, there is no end of suffering, nor a path, because there is no path, there is no knowledge, there is no gaining of enlightenment, only the destruction of obstructions.'

"The Bodhisattva Avalokitesvara has no obstruction to his mind, he follows his heart without mental hindrance because he has no obstruction, he has no fear, no fright, no fight. By inverting his dreams he goes far beyond confused imagination and has become free. Buddhas of the past, present and future by thus understanding have attained enlightenment and freedom. This understanding can truly protect one from suffering. Therefore you too should understand, only when all is going, going, going, going beyond, when every word of truth is going, only then there is a beginning of understanding.

Udana 8.1: go beyond

When Gotama was staying near Savatthi at Jeta's Grove, at Anathapindika's monastery, he was instructing and encouraging the monks there with a Dharma talk on unbinding. Noticing that all the monks were attentive, focused with their entire awareness, Gotama said,

The cessation of suffering is discerned by understanding there is that which is not understood, not made, not imagined, not fabricated by mind, not perceived through self, that which neither is begun nor ends; there is truth that exists independent of direct perception or communication. Bring an ending to your pain and pleasure, bring an end to your suffering and unbind, and you will discover what remains. You must go beyond the suffering, the origin of suffering, the cessation of suffering, and even the path leading to the ending of that suffering to gain a beginning of understanding.

The diamond

One day when Gotama lived in Sravasti, in Jeta's Grove, in the garden of Anathapindika, with more than 1,250 monks and nuns, many

Bodhisattvas, pious laity, and numerous great beings, he had returned from collecting alms in Sravasti and finished his meal. He put away his bowl and cloak, and washed his feet. Then he sat down on a seat prepared for him, and crossing his legs, holding his body upright and was mindfully attentive to the crowd who walked about him three times counterclockwise, saluting him, and sat down.

At that time, Subhuti came into that assembly and, sitting down, instantly rose from his seat. He put his robe over his shoulder, and knelt on his right knee, and bent his folded hands to Gotama, begging Gotama to explain proper view for the Bodhisattva?

Gotama answered, Subhuti, someone who has set out in the vehicle of a Bodhisattva should produce a thought in this manner: "as many beings as there are in this universe of beings, all these I must lead to freedom from suffering. And yet, though innumerable beings have thus been led to freedom, no being at all has been led to freedom." Why? For should in the Bodhisattva a notion of "being" occur, that Bodhisattva could not be called a Bodhisattva – for the notion of self has taken place through the notion of other beings."

Gotama continued, "moreover, Subhuti, a Bodhisattva who gives anything could not be a Bodhisattva: for when a gift is given that is identifiable, tangible, measurable, it is subject to suffering. Is it possible to measure the extent of the south, the west, the east, or north? Is it possible to measure the distance of downward, or upward? Even so, what a Bodhisattva gives is not easy to measure. What do you think, Subhuti, can a Tathagata be directly identified and observed?"

Subhuti replied that a Tathagata could not, that a Tathagata could only be indirectly identified and observed.

Gotama said, "indeed, wherever there is something to directly identify, or something which is unidentified, there would be a fraudulent Tathagata."

Subhuti asked, "will there be any beings in that dark, last epoch of the Dharma who will understand this nature of truth?"

Gotama answered that there would be. "Even at that time there will be Bodhisattvas who are will understand the nature of truth – and there will be many who glimpse at truth. By gaining even a moment of serenity from their understanding, they will honor all the innumerable Buddhas: they will have no perception of self, they will have no perception of a being, no perception of a soul, nor any perception of a person and identity. They will perceive the Dharma by perceiving Nodharma - by Noperception they will perceive Nonperception. They will not seize and attach to a self, a being, a soul, a person or anything at all; they will not attach to Dharma – and will not attach to Nodharma. They will understand that which is hidden through inference and, like discarding the raft used to cross a stream, will not forsake the Dharma prematurely or too late, but will still more readily forsake Nodharma."

Gotama asked, "what do you think, Subhuti, is there any Dharma which the Tathagata has fully known as 'the utmost, right and perfect enlightenment,' or is there any Dharma which the Tathagata has ever once demonstrated?"

Subhuti replied: "No, not that I know of."

Gotama asked Subhuti, "and why is this? The Dharma which the Tathagata has fully known or demonstrated cannot be directly talked about, it cannot be directly demonstrated, it is neither a Dharma nor a Nodharma."

Gotama said, "some people give gifts to exalt what they venerate as holy; they would fill a world with worlds and give those worlds in pious devotion. But if they would simply understand the Dharma as I have, they would truly honor all the innumerable Buddhas; if they would teach as I have, they would earn greater honor than a person who gave all the world."

Gotama asked, "what do you think, Subhuti, does it occur to a Tathagata, 'this Dharma is mine?' Of course not, Dharma cannot be possessed or earned – no more than anything which is seen, heard, tasted, smelled, touched or known can become yours. Freedom from suffering cannot be yours, though you can be free from suffering. Such Nofreedom is called Arhat, it is the embodiment of Nodharma – a Tathagata is not an Arhat, for this would require that the Tathagata be identifiable, have identity, to be. There is Nodharma that I have learned. There is that which exists independent of what is directly perceived."

Gotama said, "there is that which the Tathagata has taught as wisdom which has gone beyond, there is that which the Tathagata has taught as not gone beyond. Subhuti, do you think that the specks of dust that exist in trillion worlds are numerous?"

Subhuti said, yes.

Gotama asked Subhuti, "but did I teach you the number of specks of dust in a trillion worlds? Did anyone? I taught you nothing of specks of dust, nor did anyone. I did not even teach you what specks of dust were – or tell you about any of the trillion worlds – yet you understood that there would be many specks of dust in a trillion worlds."

Gotama asked, "Subhuti, did you even consider how many specks of dust there were in this world – let alone the trillions of worlds there are until I asked the question? I taught you about specks of dust and worlds by Noteaching of Nospecks and Noworlds. So it is that I teach Nodharma. Subhuti, a person can renounce the world and all their belongings, all their attachments, all their bad habits as many times as there are grains of sand in the Ganges, but it would do less good than to understand - if only for a moment - the nature of truth, and to truly perceive reality."

Gotama said, "in that distant time, the last epoch of the Dharma, there will be profound understanding.

Those who by my form did see me,
And those who followed me by voice
Wrong the efforts they engaged in,
Me those people will not see.
From the Dharma should one see the Buddhas,
From the Dharmabodies comes their guidance.
Yet Dharma's true nature cannot be discerned,
And no one can be conscious of it as an object.

Someone honorable does not acquire honor, does not gain honor. Honor cannot be given or received. Whoever says that the Tathagata goes or comes, stands, sits or lies down – they do not understand my teaching. The Tathagata is called one who has not gone anywhere, nor has come from anywhere, acquired nothing, given nothing."

Gotama asked, "Subhuti, has the Tathagata ever taught a view of being, a view of a living soul, a view of identity? Only Noview has been taught by the Tathagata. No beliefs have been taught, only that there are beliefs – and such beliefs may be let go. A Bodhisattva should know all Dharma. And by this knowledge not perceive the Dharma. And if a Bodhisattva should teach the Dharma – it should be illuminated, but not revealed: as stars shine but do not guide, as by a fault of vision one sees, as a lamp illuminates but does not show, as a mock show demonstrates but does not teach; like a dew drop, or like a bubble, like a dream, like a lightning flash, or a cloud – such is right view."

Anguttara Nikaya 5.41: the price of honor

Gotama understood what was troubling Anathapindika, and said,

There is a use for wealth, Anathapindika. Consider the righteous benefits that can be obtained from wealth, Anathapindika. But first wealth must first be earned rightly. If the wealth is earned rightly, wealth can provide many benefits.

Wealth can maintain and enable not only to the self, but family, servants, assistants, friends, partners, and the entire community free of want, in contentment.

Wealth can also be used against disasters, both within the household and community, arising from fire, or flood, wars, or kings, or even thieves and hateful heirs, or similar disasters.

Wealth can be used to purchase offerings to guests, relatives, nobles, the household's gods or even the dead, all those who should be honored by gifts.

Wealth can also be spent through generosity and charity, through selfless gifts to righteous men and women, or for righteous causes.

When wealth is spent in these ways, a wealthy person has no regret, even if they deplete their entire fortune, for they will have obtained all the righteous benefit they could from their wealth. And, even if their wealth increases by spending it in these ways, they will still feel no remorse, because they will continue to obtain the full righteous benefit they can from their wealth.

Anathapindika, it is possible to enjoy your wealth without remorse, if you spend it righteously. Do not hold onto your wealth or attach to it. Support your family and friends, your associates in business and in the community; give generous offerings to your guests and all those you would honor; provide for righteous men and women, and righteous causes; protect your community against all disaster. Being thus established in my teaching, you will not only feel no remorse, but will enjoy using your wealth to obtain the greatest benefit from it.

When wealth is lost, to bad fortune or bad management, it is gone. But wealth spent righteously has purchased that which cannot ever be lost.

You might try to save your wealth, deep underground, at the water line, thinking, "when need or duty arises, this will provide for my needs, for bail if I am wrongfully arrested, for my rescue if I am robbed, in case of debt, famine or accidents." And so a reserve fund is stashed away, seemingly prudently. But no matter how well it's stored, deep underground or in a safe, no matter how prudently it is saved into, it will never be enough to serve you at your time of need. The fund gets shifted from its place, or one's memory gets confused; or – unseen –water serpents make off with it, spirits steal it, or hateful heirs run off with it. Or it gets spent on frivolous things. Or perhaps the need is too great and it is simply not enough.

But when you spend your wealth righteously, that honor it purchases can never be taken, and will always be enough.

Therefore, spend your wealth righteously, with a sense of conviction, attentive to whom you are giving it and their needs. Give with an empathetic heart, selflessly, without adversely affecting yourself or others who depend on you.

Anguttara Nikaya 5.43: do not pray

Anathapindika had gone to Gotama, and after he had sat down Gotama said to him,

What is desirable cannot be obtained by prayers or wishes. Long life and health is welcome, agreeable, pleasant, but hard to obtain. Beauty and comfort is welcome, agreeable, pleasant, but hard to obtain. Contentment and happiness is welcome, agreeable, pleasant, but hard to obtain. Power and status is welcome, agreeable, pleasant, but hard to obtain. A better life is welcome, agreeable, pleasant, but hard to obtain.

If what was desirable could be obtained simply by prayers or wishes, who among us would lack what we desire? It is not fitting for one of my students to pray or wish for their desires. If something is desired, they will simply understand how to obtain it by understanding its nature and causes, and work to follow the path leading to what they desire.

Samyutta Nikaya 55.22: the leaning tree

When Gotama was staying among the Sakyans near Kapilavatthu in Nigrodha's Park, Mahanama the Sakyan went to Gotama and said, "while I pass through Kapilavatthu in the evening after visiting you and your monks, the streets are so crowded and the people so rich and prosperous that the lessons I just heard become muddled in my head from distraction. I am sometimes afraid I will die when a runaway elephant or horse threatens to trample me, or a chariot nearly runs me over. At times like those, I even forget you, and the monks, and the Dharma I learned. I am concerned that if I were to die in Kapilavatthu I will die badly."

Gotama comforted him, "don't fear, Mahanama, your death will not be a bad one. Even so distracted and afraid, you will unbind from your suffering because you have confidence in me as your teacher; you have confidence in the Dharma I teach; you have confidence that the Dharma I have taught, if practiced well, methodically, may be mastered, and that those who have mastered it in my Sangha are worthy of respect; you are endowed with virtues that I – and all my monks – find appealing."

Gotama comforted him more, "suppose, Mahanama, that a tree was leaning and inclining toward the east, if its root were cut, which way would it fall?"

"In whatever direction it was leaning and inclining, Sir," said Mahanama.

Gotama comforted Mahanama, "it is just so, it is the same way, Mahanama, when someone inclines toward liberation dies. They do not die badly."

Anguttara Nikaya 8.53: Gotami the nun

Gotama's mother had died in childbirth. His adoptive mother was his aunt, and loved him so that she gave her two natural children to nurses, and nursed Gotama herself.

Almost immediately after he had attained his enlightenment, his adoptive mother, and aunt, Mahapajapati Gotami, asked Gotama for ordination as a nun. She would have been the first nun. To her surprise, Gotama refused, and then left for Vesali. Many women were discouraged: if he refused to ordain even his aunt and adoptive mother, were there to be no nuns at all?

But Mahapajapati Gotami was undaunted. She cut off her hair and put on the robes of a monk, and encouraged a large number of women to do the same. They followed her adoptive son to Vesali on foot.

Upon arrival, she repeated her request to be ordained to Ananda, who agreed to intercede with her adoptive son on her behalf. He respectfully questioned the Buddha:

"Sir, are women capable of attaining enlightenment?"

"They are, Ananda," said the Buddha.

"If that is so, Sir, it would be good if women could be allowed to join the Sangha, and even ordained as nuns. It would be good if Mahapajapati Gotami would be allowed to join the Sangha and become ordained as a nun."

"Ananda, I cannot allow Mahapajapati Gotami to join the Sangha or become a nun, for she already has joined the Sangha and became a nun. She only must now only perfect her training."

Ananda shared what Gotama said with Gotami, and Gotami was encouraged. Gotami then went to her adoptive son, the Buddha Gotama, and asked that he teach her the Dharma in brief.

Gotama again refused her. He said to her, "but Gotami, you already know the Dharma, the Vinaya, my instructions? You know some things lead to the cessation of suffering, you know to seek dispassion, disattachment, modesty, contentment, disentaglement, seclusion, persistence, unburdening ..."

Majjhima Nikaya 12: extraordinary powers

Once, when Gotama was living at Vasali in the grove outside the city to the west, Sunakkhatta, left the Dharma and the Discipline, saying "Gotama has no superhuman states, no supernatural distinction in knowledge and vision. He teaches a Dharma of reasoning and logic, follows a line of inquiry chosen by him toward the destruction of suffering. When he teaches the Dharma to anyone, it only leads to the destruction of suffering."

Sariputta heard Sunakkhatta, he went to Gotama and said what he heard. Gotama assured Sariputta, "Sariputta, Sunakkhatta is angry, and his words are spoken out of anger. But thinking to discredit me he actually praises me. Though he understands the truth, he will never understand that this signifies I am accomplished, enlightened, perfected in my knowledge and conduct. He will never perceive the superhuman and supernatural power of logic and reasoning."

"Sariputta, a Tathagata such as myself has ten powers. A Tathagata understands what is possible as possible and what is impossible as impossible. A Tathagata understands nature of causational reaction: what is has happened because of what occurred in the past, and what will happen is because of what is done now. A Tathagata understands the ways leading to all destinations, understanding the world with its many and different elements. A Tathagata understands how beings have become inclined toward different actions, and the nature and disposition of other beings and persons. A Tathagata understands the jhanas, liberations, concentrations and attainments. A Tathagata recollects all their manifold past lives, and perceives the passing away and reappearing of other beings. By realization of direct knowledge, a Tathagata abides free of suffering."

Samyutta Nikaya 5.2, Majjhima Nikaya 44: self sacrifice (sacrifice of identity)

The nun Soma was meditating in the Blind Man's Grove near Savatthi when Mara saw her there. Embodying himself as delusion, Mara approached her and spoke to her quietly. "In the Blind Man's grove, you cannot attain what requires sight; women should not reach, for they lack sufficient wisdom."

Soma was quick to respond to Mara, "Am I a woman? For someone who understands the Dharma, the question never arises, am I man or woman? Or, am I anything at all? I understand the Dharma with a well composed mind, and you, Mara, may talk to me as much as you like."

Mara then vanished.

(Mara is another name for Maya)

From gender identity to political identity, from nationality to religion, we self-identify – and this results in suffering.

When Gotama was staying in Rajagaha, in the bamboo grove of the squirrels' sanctuary, Visakha the layman went to Dhammadinna the nun and asked her to explain what Gotama meant when he referred to self-identification?

She said, pleasure can be generally understood to be whatever is gratifying – to body, mind or heart. Pain can be generally understood to be whatever is displeasing to body mind or heart. Both result in suffering, discontentment, distress: what displeases is discontenting, distressing, and must be suffered – and what is pleasurable cannot be sustained, and this is displeasing, distressing and must be suffered.

Self identification results when there is desire for pleasure and aversion to pain, especially the desire for becoming and the aversion to unbecoming. This results in an individual attaching to beliefs regarding their form, feelings, and other constructed beliefs – the way these forms were, are, will be, should be, shouldn't be, can't be, won't be, aren't, weren't.

Such belief results in the individual assuming that their body is their self, or that their self possesses form. They assume that their feelings are their self, or that their self possesses feelings. That what they perceive, think and believe are all their self, or that their self possesses such attributes.

Understanding that such things are not the self permits an awareness of the process of identification, and that identification results in the suffering which the individual was attempting to avoid: whatever was, is or will be is impermanent, and subject to unbecoming – and rebecoming. All that began must end, and all that ends must begin – as such beginning and ending causes displeasure, discontentment, distress, suffering, then the individual should consider that beliefs also change. And most importantly that beliefs can be let go of entirely.

Identification can be ceased. The suffering of identification can cease.

Anguttara Nikaya 3.62: danger

There are dangers which can separate a mother and her child.

Most people think that such dangers are those seen in great fire, or flood, or war, or some kind of crime. And indeed there may come a time when a great fire breaks out. The fire might burn a village, or a town or even a city. When it is burning, a mother there might not be able to get to her child, and the child unable to get to its mother. And it is true that sometimes a cloud forms, and from its rain a great flood of water is produced, flooding villages, towns and even cities. During this flood, a mother might not be able to get to her child, and a child might not be able to get to its mother. And sometimes during war or crime, enemies invade a home, or a region, or even a nation. After they take power and control, they even surround the lands about the home, the region, or the nation, occupying even the countryside. In such times, mothers and children are frequently separated.

Yet those dangers are not always separating mothers and their children. There are also times when during fire, flood or invasion, a mother might get to her child, or the child can get to the mother – despite the dangers. Much can be done by mother and child against such dangers, and often, mother and child get their wish in regard to the separation during these dangers to be reunited after the danger has passed. Indeed, sometimes such dangers can even reunify mother and child.

But there are dangers from which mothers and children always are separated: aging, illness and death.

Never has a mother gotten her wish in regard to a child who is aging, "I am aging, but may my child not age." And never has a child gotten its wish in regard to its mother who is aging, "I am aging, but may my mother not age." By age, mother and child will be forever separated. Never has a mother or child gotten their wish to not be separated by illness, or death.

Yet by right view, right resolve, right speech, right action, right livelihood, right effort, right mindfulness and right concentration, the mother and child need not suffer from their separation, even if they are to remain separated. Mother and child both must strive for this abandoning and overcoming of their suffering.

Indeed, without these eight practices for overcoming suffering, mother and child will not only certainly suffer, but will certainly become separated – even without fire, flood or war, aging, illness or death.

Observe that families are frequently separated without fire, flood, war, crime, aging, illness or death by wrong views, wrong resolves, wrong speech, wrong action, wrong livelihood, wrong effort, wrong mindfulness, and wrong concentration. These are far more dangerous than fire, flood, criminals or invading armies, far more dangerous than aging, illness or death.

The death of the Buddha Gotama

The Buddha Gotama said that most of the things in the world are subject to change, but there are in this world four things that do not change: the permanence of suffering, the origin of suffering, the cessation of suffering, the way leading to the cessation of suffering. He said that these should be understood, and the understanding of these is necessary to liberate yourself from suffering.

Further, he encouraged his students: they could personally understand these truths through direct experience!

But permanence was and is still a difficult thing to comprehend. The Buddha attempted to explain the permanence of the truth these four permanent things, and the truth of all that he taught, by saying they were so permanent that they would outlast even the memory of his own existence…and told a story of a famous drum.

Long before he died, the Buddha said, there once was a time when the Dasarahas had a large drum the called "the Summoner." It could be heard for 11 miles! But, it grew old and the wood split.

So, the Dasarahas inserted a peg in it, and kept playing. But it then it could only be heard for 10 miles. It kept splitting, and they kept inserting pegs into it, and Summoner kept getting quieter, until the time came when Summoner's original wooden body had disappeared and only a conglomeration of pegs remained and you couldn't hear Summoner if it were played behind a curtain!

He said that in the same way, there would come a time in the future people would not listen when the teachings are read, and won't read them when they are written. Even monks and nuns will not set their hearts upon the lessons, and won't regard the lessons as worth knowing or mastering. In that distant future, people will listen when the works of poets are recited, and will read great works of rhetoric and elegance. To these works they will set their hearts, and regard them as worth knowing and mastering.

The Buddha said that this is how his words will disappear, his lessons will be forgotten. All things are impermanent.

Against those future times, said the Buddha, you should train yourself first to listen to the lessons of the Buddha when they are spoken, and read them when they are written. "This we will do!" swore the monks attending the lecture of the Buddha.

When the Buddha died at the age of 80, he repeated this lesson. At the moment of his death, he warned all his students so would die also all things except the truth of what he taught. "Now, strive for your own liberation with diligence," were his final words.

~   ~   ~   ~   ~   ~   ~   ~   ~

Gotama had sickened from the meal of meat soup that Cunda had given him and was dying. Gotama said, "Please, Ananda, comfort Cunda against his remorse. He killed me, but did no wrong."

Ananda sadly acknowledged the man born his cousin, who had been his King, his lifelong friend and said, "I shall, my Lord." Gotama then said, "come, Ananda, let us cross to the farther bank of the Hirannavati, and go to the Sala Grove of the Mallas family, near Kusinara." When they arrived, Gotama asked Ananda to prepare for him a couch between the twin sala trees. "I am weary, Ananda, and want to lie down." "So be it, Lord," said Ananda. Gotama laid upon the couch in the Lion position, one foot upon the other.

Gotama, the King, son of Kings, at length said to Ananda, "Ananda, I shall die very soon, and I wish my body to be burned like the noble King I have become." He then fell deep in contemplation. As he lay there, the salas blossomed, flowered and dropped their petals upon him, the stars themselves began to fall to the sound of distant music in the heavens, and the smell of sandalwood and other sweet incense filled the air while Ananda stood, ready at service.

The flowers disturbed Gotama from his meditation, and he smiled, weakly. "Ananda, it seems the salas flower out of season for me. Yet I wish you to understand that the honor these trees do for me is nothing against the reverence a monk or nun or layperson would do me by living rightly by my teachings." Ananda bowed low, and vowed, "Lord, we shall do as you have taught and abide by the Dharma, live rightly by the Dharma and walk in the way of the Dharma."

During the night, all the people and other beings that could come came to visit Gotama and paid their final respects. In the procession, Ananda slipped away to the nearby monastery. At the gate, Ananda stood quietly in the night. Then he leaned against the doorpost of the gate. Then he fell to his knees and wept. It was at that moment a monk quietly approached him, and told him that Gotama had called for him. Ananda rushed back.

When Ananda approached Gotama, Gotama sat up weakly and said, "enough, Ananda! Do not grieve! Have I not taught from the very beginning that with all that is dear and beloved there must be change, separation, and severance? Of that which is born, come into being, compounded, and subject to decay, how could anyone say: 'May it not come to dissolution?' There can be no such state of things." Gotama comforted his friend and servant. "Now for a long time, Ananda, you have served me with loving-kindness in deed, word, and thought, graciously, pleasantly, with a whole heart and beyond measure. Great good have you gathered, Ananda! Now you should put forth energy, and soon you too will be free."

Gotama then addressed those who had gathered to him, "I wish you to look at Ananda. Ananda has good and superlative qualities. If laypeople or a company of monks and nuns see Ananda, they become joyful on seeing him; and if he then speaks to them of the Dharma, they are made joyful by his discourse; and when he becomes silent, they are disappointed. In the future, when I am gone, do not say that you are masterless, for you shall have Ananda. Though he has not yet attained enlightenment, he is already like a noble King."

Ananda then realized that his King was dying in the wilds, a place he believed unbefitting such a nobleman as he was. He suggested to Gotama that he allow himself to be removed to a large and noble city, where he might die attended by great men and women, with reverence proper to his nobility. Gotama said, "do not weep that I should die in this mean place, the middle of the jungle, away from society. In this same place, long ago, there ruled a noble King by the name of Maha Sudassana, it was his royal capital of Kusavati. Kusavati, Ananda, resounded unceasingly day and night with trumpeting elephants, neighing horses, rattling of chariots, beating of drums and tambourines, music, song, cheers, the clapping of hands, and cries of 'Eat, drink, and be merry!' I would not call it a mean place, something of its greatness remains. And something of my greatness will remain when I, too, die."

Gotama grew weaker and the Malla family were called by him, and given custody over his remains, for he was dying in their grove. At that moment a wandering ascetic named Subhadda came to learn from Gotama. Subhadda asked to be admitted to the Buddha's presence, and was directed to Ananda, who refused him because Gotama was dying and there were so many disciples that were ahead of him in line. Three times Subhadda insisted before Gotama himself heard Ananda deny him. Gotama then asked that Subhadda be admitted and admonished Ananda, telling him that all who come to learn should be admitted.

Subhadda thanked the Buddha and knelt down beside where the Buddha lay, and, after being instructed, took vows, becoming the last disciple taught by Gotama himself. Gotama then asked that Ananda impose the greatest penalty upon Channa. "I shall, Lord, but do not know what is the greatest penalty I can impose upon a monk or layperson is?" asked Ananda. Gotama said, "let him say and do what he will, but none should converse with him, exhort him, or admonish him." With Ananda in his usual place of attendance, Gotama gave his final lesson, and then, after asking if anyone desired any clarification or further learning from him before he died (no one did), resumed his meditation and died.

After a week of mourning, the Malla family asked Ananda what they should do with the body of Gotama? Remembering what his master had said, Ananda told them, "burn it, like a noble King's body."

~   ~   ~   ~   ~   ~   ~   ~

Many came to visit the tomb, and asked how their King had died. Ananda explained that Gotama had sickened from the meal of meat soup that Cunda had given him. Ananda said Gotama had said to him, "Please, Ananda, comfort Cunda against his remorse. He killed me, but did no wrong."

The Buddha Gotama had arrived in Pava while wandering with a large community of monks, and stayed in the mango grove of Cunda the metalworker. When Cunda heard that the Buddha was staying in his mango grove, he visited the Buddha, and Gotama taught him the Dharma. Grateful, Cunda, invited the Buddha to dine with him the next day, with all the community of monks.

Cunda was busy the entire night preparing a delicious feast of meat, and when it was ready, he announced to the Buddha that the meal was ready. Then Gotama, early in the morning, carried his bowl and robes and went together with the community of monks to Cunda's home. On arrival, he sat down on the seat prepared for him. Understanding the significance of the meal prepared for him, that it would be his last and fatal, when he was seated and the meal ready to be served, he said to Cunda, "Cunda, serve me with the meat soup you have had prepared, and the community of monks with the other food you have had prepared."

Cunda obeyed, "as you say, Lord." When the food was served as Gotama had directed and everyone was eating and full, Gotama said, "Cunda, bury the remaining meat soup in a pit. I don't see anyone in the world who could eat it and develop a healthy change, except myself." Cunda, puzzled, obeyed. "as you say, Lord," and buried the meat soup. When he returned, the Buddha again instructed him in the Dharma, and left.

Shortly after leaving, there arose in the Buddha serious illness. He passed tremendous quantities of blood, and had intense and deadly pains throughout his body. In his sudden illness, he fell. But the Buddha Gotama endured his misery, mindful and alert.

Gotama had sickened from the meal of meat soup that Cunda had given him and was dying. Gotama said, "Please, Ananda, comfort Cunda against his remorse. He killed me, but did no wrong." Ananda sadly acknowledged his worldly king and cousin, his childhood playmate, his friend and said, "I shall, my Lord."

The Buddha in his misery laid down, and begged Ananda for water. Ananda, worried for the health of the Buddha, hurried to the river. But he did not return with water, saying "Lord, just now 500 carts have passed through. The small river – cut by the wheels – flows turbid and disturbed. But the Kukuta river is not far away, with pristine, cool, healthful water, with restful banks, refreshing to you. There you will drink potable water and cool your fever," and urged his Lord to come there.

But the Buddha a second and a third time denied Ananda, and begged Ananda, "please fetch me some water. I am thirsty. I will drink the water there." Ananda, at last, obeyed, "as you say, Lord." He took a bowl and went to the river. To his surprise, the turbid river now flowed pristine, clear and undisturbed. He brought the water back to the Buddha, and Gotama drank his last drink of water.

With the water, he then grew strong enough to cross the small river, and bathe in it. Upon the other side, he grew very weak, and, traveling a little further, directed Ananda to make for him a bed to die upon in a Sala grove, and to burn his body as the noble King.

After Gotama's hot fever burned out and the cold corpse was cremated as befitting a noble King, Ananda kept his duty and traveled again to see Cunda, so he might perform his duty, and deliver to him the Buddha's message. "Cunda, the Buddha Gotama wished you to be comforted against your regret. You gave to him his last meal with pure heart, and for such a giving person, merit increases. Cunda, a person with self restraint amasses no hatred. One who is skillful leaves evil behind and thereby ends his sins, his aggression, aversion, desire and ignorance. Thus freed, he gains the right of self-awakening, and will enjoy life, beauty, happiness, bliss, the sovereignty of a noble king."

~   ~   ~   ~   ~   ~   ~   ~

Cunda remembered how Gotama had said to him, "Cunda, bury the remaining meat soup in a pit. I don't see anyone in the world who could eat it and develop a healthy change, except myself." Cunda, puzzled, had obeyed. When he returned, the Buddha again instructed him in the Dharma...

"Lord, how many kinds of Buddhists are there in the world?" Asked Cunda of Gotama.

"Four, Cunda. Let me explain. There is the one who is victor of the path, who, has his second arrow of suffering removed, delighting in his freedom from desire and aversion, his freedom from ignorance and hatred, the victor of the path is a noble King. There is another who, knowing foremost, shows and analyzes the Dharma, a sage, a destroyer of doubt, and is a teacher of the path. The third lives by the well-taught path, the path of Dharma, associating without blame or fight, at peace, a companion on the path. But the fourth is a fraud of the other three, self-asserting, a corrupter, intrusive, deceitful, unrestrained, chaff, going about in disguise, this fourth corrupts the path."

Gotama then answered the question unasked upon Cunda's mind. "Don't worry, Cunda. Anyone can discern a corrupter from the other three, even without knowing much about the Dharma: a corrupter does not merely teach incorrectly, does not merely live incorrectly, but performs services that are inappropriate for themselves to do for rewards that are inappropriate for themselves to earn, and works against those who live by Dharma, encouraging others against them in hatred."

"Cunda, a Buddhist conquers their suffering. And helps others to do so through loving kindness, the compassion of friendship, as a noble King, a teacher, a companion on the path."

Shortly after leaving Cunda, there arose in the Buddha serious illness. He passed tremendous quantities of blood, and had intense and deadly pains throughout his body. In this sudden illness, he fell, and knew he was going to die.

He asked to be buried as a noble King, a victor of the path.

Editor's note: When the Buddha was born, his mother died in childbirth, holding onto the limbs of a tree to ease birth, shaking loose the flowers in her contractions and death spasms; these continued to fall on the newly born child. It is poetic that at his death, Gotama's dying spasms also shook loose flowers.

Theragatha 17.3: eulogy

Ananda, grieving for Gotama, said, "tonight, all directions are obscure, none of the teachings are clear. For one whose friend has passed away, one whose teacher is gone for good, though I am now surrounded by friends, there is no other friend that will do. I only reflect that all my old friends are dead. I do not feel I fit in with all these new and young friends. So tonight I shall remember, reflect and muse alone, like a bird who has gone to roost."

Ananda continued his eulogy. "When he died, there was terror, and my hair stood up on end. He was a virtuous, wise man –"

And right then, suddenly, understanding his friend and teacher was just a man, and was dead, Ananda, the attendant, understood the impermanence of all things, and extinguished his self to become enlightened.

Ananda said, "I heard 82,000 teachings from the Buddha Gotama, 2,000 more from his disciples. I had memorized and learned 84,000 lessons in total. Yet for all I heard, I understood nothing until right now. I was like a blind man, holding a lamp."

And so Ananda inwardly collected his mind, and began to teach...

Excerpt from the Khandoga Upanishad

Meditate on the syllable Om. This syllable is sometimes called the Udgitha because a portion of the Samaveda (the Udgitha) is sung beginning with Om. The nature of all beings of the earth, all material and matter, animate and inanimate, all speech, the essence of the Rigveda and Samaveda can be understood by meditating on this one syllable: by understanding that speech coarises with breath, you can understand the codependent nature of suffering. The meditation of Om is one of permission, of permitting things to coexist, coarise, coterminate: just as when two people come together in friendship and love, they would naturally fulfil each other's desire, so does breath and speech fulfill the other's purpose - and by understanding this, you can fulfill your purpose. By such meditation we understand the nature of sacrifice. Om can be used to understand co-conditoinality. Breath, voice and mouth are used to shape the word, without any one of these, the word is not formed: like fire emerges naturally when spark, fuel and air coincide, victory in yoga results upon the conditioning of success.

The Priest gives an order and says "Om!" When the Hotri Priest recites, they say "Om!" When the Udgartri Priest sings, they say "Om!" Om! Om! Om! All because of the importance of meditating on that one syllable. Whoever knows the meaning of Om, having meditated on it and understood it, and whoever does not understand Om - both would perform the same sacrifice. But whoever does not understand Om would lack benefits the sacrifice would bring. This is why it is said there is a secret meaning of Om.

Week 12

SUMMARY.

Final instruction: Satsangha, going forth, teaching. Advanced Class: Teacher training. Annapurna, animal sacrifice (vegetarianism).

- Students come prepared to teach a short lesson, and are organized into a Sadhana Ashrama, where at regular meetings they share the duties of leading instruction, training, debate and practice and prepare and organize performances of Dharma.
- An introduction to vegetarianism is made.
- Students contribute to annapurna. Students are encouraged to beg foods for their vegetarian annapurna performance. Each student brings enough food for themselves.

Satsangha

There are many reasons for which socialization are undertaken, and this results in numerous types of relationships. The satsangha, the association of true people, is not undertaken for a particular purpose, but emerges as a result of a common Dharma within people. Here, a common purpose and practice unites (if only for a short time). Sharing, and caring, for each other results.

The wider satsangha of the world, in the blogosphere and world wide web, on youtube, and at your places of work, and living, to greater or lesser degree are similar associations. We seek the company of friends who can help, who can support, who can share, who can give, who can receive.

Loka, Hatha Yoga!

At this Ashrama of Sadhana, at this moment of effort and accomplishment, we become prepared to journey on. Discipline is undertaken to accomplish a goal, and we would live and work together.

Though the meeting places and times cannot be conveniently published in a book format, if you did not attend this class, please contact Loka Hatha Yoga. We would meet with you to learn from you, and perform what duties we share together.

Going forth: you are ready to begin

No human has ever accomplished sufficient training as to utterly defeat their aggression, desire or ignorance: it is by continued practice and training that we maintain self-control. Even a well trained horse will wilder if permitted unrestrained freedom, and if permitted loose reigns will sooner or later determine its own direction. Even farmland cultivated for millennia will wilder if spared the plow and fallowed too long, even the freshly tilled field sprouts weeds. Even a long-occupied region will rebel if permitted to assert its own traditions, and retains its distinctive identity. Don't you know your nature by now to think better against the possibility of final victory?

What then is the victory blow? How do you fulfill your vows? Where is the safety and refuge in this world?

Walking barefoot across the world, the sharp stones and thorns will destroy your feet. Do you stay indoors? Or venture out to the hard world? Venturing out, would you lay down cloth to protect yourself? Where would you find enough cloth to cover the surface of this planet? Only obtain enough cloth to cover the soles of your feet, continually laying the cloth between your foot and the ground with each step, and your feet will not be destroyed, even should you wander the entire hard world.

Who can utterly destroy all their aggression, desire or ignorance? Who needs to? No one has ever accomplished such a thing, nor has any such thing been required..

Does one blot out the sun to find relief in the summer heat - or find shelter inside a building, in a cool river, or under an umbrella? Would you imagine malice in the weather where there is only your own negligence? It is your fault, and yours alone, if you get sunburned. The sun's nature is to burn you. As will all light, and heat, all fire.

And should you burn, remember it is likely you will recover. It is sometimes worth a little sunburn to enjoy the benefits of daylight. The world is a dangerous place and you may feel unsafe, but you are safe enough. Do you truly need a refuge?

You may indeed feel underpracticed, undertrained, but you are ready enough. Svaha! Go forth from this place of safety. Is this not what you have endeavored to achieve? Is this not the accomplishment of your goal? Not the safety of a prison, but the strength to endure the world in peace. Enough! Go! Extinguish your flame!

For one who has learned self-restraint, there is no need to fear others from inspiring anger or any other undesired emotion, from inspiring your own aggression, from inspiring your own desire, or causing your own ignorance. Consider "who would restrain this mind of mine but myself?" Like a horse, like a field, like some oppressed people, would you actually want another to restrain you and cultivate you and protect you? You need no chaperone, nor want one. What greater use is refuge than a friend could be to someone like you? Seek friendship, if you would be forever safe.

Thus you should train and practice yourself in alertness. Examine again and again the condition of your body and mind. Practice jnana. Then do not hesitate to do what is necessary: it does no good to be aware of a problem and then do nothing about it. Do the sick receive benefit merely by reading medical texts? Are the recipes in a cookbook delicious and wholesome to merely read? Why did you undertake this training? For what purpose do you practice?

Without intending to become angry, people become angry. Without intending to become disheartened, or even depressed, people become cold, and hating. There is no intention to emotion, though there is purpose to it: these are merely biological functions, like defecation, or breathing.

Yet some will resist or suppress their emotions, thinking by resistance or suppressing they need not act on them and be free of them. This rarely is successful. Upon feeling and thinking, even after resisting or suppressing, some people act on these thoughts and feelings, others do not. Know it is by training and practice in tolerance of these sensations and thoughts that one learns to not act without intention. Do not let the pain or pleasure of a thought or feeling compel you to do what you know is unnecessary or unuseful.

Mistakes will happen. No one is strong enough to avoid mistakes. You will make mistakes. Yet it is an error to conclude that mistakes occur only because of the force of external conditions, and not to consider our own insufficient strength as the cause. When you err, know it is your own fault. Then you can grow stronger by your error.

Emotions and thoughts are biological facts, but are as random and directionless as any environmental effect: for they are independent of the will, even as the mind is independent of the body. Our senses are independent of the interpretation of them: distrust what you see, hear, smell, touch, and taste. And especially what you think and feel. Practice jnana, and you will be aware of this necessity, and more. There is a necessity to using logic to evaluate and intend before acting.

Be aware, of all the dangers to be wary of, thoughts and feelings are the greatest. Of these, anger and hatred are the strongest. But it is not necessary to suppress them to bring them under control: it is not necessary to avoid anger or hatred, in yourself or others. They arise, and last a while, and then dissipate - as all thoughts and feelings do. No asana can be held indefinitely. Permit yourself to feel them, intensely, exhaust them, see their illusionary nature. Practice and train in forgiveness, in love, so that these become reflexive to anger and hatred, so that you become accustomed to understanding anger and hatred fade, and will be better inclined to naturally advantage yourself of the wisdom that comes subsequent to any extreme thought or feeling.

There is always shame in anger and hatred: it is by anger and hatred we break what we love and think precious, it is by anger and hatred we give offense to those we love. It is by anger and hatred we cause many forms of disrespect. How can there be any honor from such dishonor?

Forgiveness and love are the means to honor. These keep the mind flexible, pliable, adaptive, and useful for what is necessary. There is also considerable strength in forgiveness and love. Sacrifice your anger and hatred, and obtain strength sufficient to withstand anger and hatred. Become strong enough for peace. Om! Shanti.

Sadness, happiness and regret, too, are dangerous, for they are deceptive, and invite ignorance: while they last, these emotions seem very real, and blind us to the reality of impermanence, and of distress. They seem to last forever, and when gone (like a dream) are quickly forgotten, so that we do not easily recall they ever were experienced, or ever ceased.

Against such delusion exercise strength in memory and foresight, understand all things begin, and end. There is pain. There is death. There is weakening, and ending. There is rebecoming. And there is greater danger in rebecoming than in re-ending, starting than stopping, continuing than pausing.

What use is there in seeking the prolonging of happiness, or the evasion of sadness? When a mistake is made, what use is there in persistent remorse? Why indulge these delusions as real?   These are all biological functions, nothing more.

When a fire enters a house, it is proper to move things away from the flames which could cause it to spread further, or even to tear down that house to protect others. By training and practice, evaluate your actions with logic to develop intention. Build fireblocks: intention and logical evaluation will protect you.

Do not act without intention, motivated by senseless thoughts and emotions which inspire aggression and ignorance and desire. Endure the pain and pleasure of these sensations: strong thoughts and emotions are painful or pleasurable, intoxicating, and addictive. Endure them long enough to logically evaluate them.

Do not react to the senseless feelings of others as if they were willful, logical, thought-through intentions, if you would not share in this intoxication.

Hold onto nothing unimportant. Enmity, jealousy, revenge, and so many other thoughts and feelings serve no useful purpose. Letting go of these, take hold of what is important.

Do not let go of important things without purpose: if you would sell something precious, do so out of urgent necessity, and then obtain a fair price for it: make sure the exchange is worthwhile, and you may enjoy what you gain by it.

Does the praise or blame or other opinions of another motivate or matter to you? Their opinions matter less than your own: both theirs and yours are tainted by bias, and are untruthful. Yet your own beliefs you may control. You may stop blaming or praising yourself. You may stop holding onto opinions. Or any other belief. You may stop seeking the praise or evading the blame of others. There is no need to praise Dharma, for it will be practiced by all sooner or later, out of urgent necessity.

To work for the benefit of all beings, that they may become aware of what is urgently necessary, and then accomplish their duty, to ensure their liberation from suffering, requires you first liberate yourself: are you not aware that there are so many others who presently work for your liberation? If you only would care for yourself, you would free them to help others who are less able than you. This is the best way to honor the efforts of your benefactors. You cannot cease until all beings are liberated: all beings together are dependent upon each other for their freedom. A bodhisattva's vow is no promise, but only an affirmation of the truth of interdependence.

Energetically, enthusiastically, exert yourself. Bear into your asanas with your heart and strength: you will find they cannot be held long and there is no long resting. This is the secret to perpetual strength: understand the nature of things is rebecoming as well as ending, that the recovery of strength is the consequence of expending it.

Remain attentive, but with the purpose of understanding; practice and train, but with the purpose of performing.

Have you not seen cattle watch their kind penned and slaughtered senselessly, while still enjoying the food laid out for them, still sleeping soundly? Surrounded as you are by death and distress, how can you sleep soundly, enjoying your meals without understanding the reason to gain and keep strength by the food is to perform your duty? Everyone dies before they feel ready. Everyone begins before they feel ready.

Will you be like that cow led to slaughter?

Do you not now see how urgent things have become? It is necessary for you to begin!

The bee does not take the whole flower back to its hive, but merely only the pollen, and only what it may carry. It is unnecessary and unuseful to take everything with you, to know everything, to know all the words there are written or said. You know enough. It is unnecessary and unuseful to know all the asanas. You know enough.

It is urgently necessary for you to begin.

Even one word well spoken is better than a thousand inappropriate phrases. Do not wait a moment longer to learn any more words. It is urgently necessary for you to begin.

There is always discomfort at awkwardness, at failure, at learning, at beginning. But as the doctor prescribes medicine which is bitter and results in terrible side effects which are tolerated because the medicine is for their wellbeing, so would we tell you to begin, and you should tolerate this discomfort as beginning is greatly to your wellbeing.

It is urgently necessary for you to begin.

Final instructions: Anguttara Nikaya 5.159

The Buddha Gotama said to Ananda, even for someone who understands the Dharma, it is not easy to teach the Dharma to others. The Dharma should only be taught when a person is able to. The teacher must teach with the thought,

I will explain how all effects have causes, and how to observe both effect and cause, for this is essential to understanding the Dharma.

I will explain those causes and effects step by step.

I will teach, motivated by compassion, not by reward.

I will teach without exalting myself, or disparaging others.

Gotama said "it is not easy to teach the Dharma, Ananda."

After Word

What is a Hindu? Am I a Hindu?
Do I believe in God?

What is a Hindu? Am I a Hindu? Do I believe in God?

Yogis know some things should not be spoken of and kept secret. The secret lies behind the door: the door is not locked; you must grow strong enough to open it – only then you will be ready to see what lies on the other side. Only then you will be ready for the secret knowledge. It does no good to tell someone what they cannot understand.

Nevertheless, I would tell you secrets today. Perhaps you are ready for them.

The Indus is a river in India, a place once known as Bharat. Hinduism is a word that its conquerors used to describe the bewildering multitude of practices undertaken there, without taking the time to understand if or even how these practices interrelated.

These practices were interrelated, as were the practices that extended from India eastward and westward: long before Christ, before Abraham, when Hindu missionaries brought Buddhism to pre-classical Greece and ancient Egypt, when they carried Ganesh as far as islands of Japan, and further, the connection in practice was neither strained nor broken. It is a practice that spans continents – and countless millennia, with living memory of those other sentient species of hominids we once lived among and fought against.

It is a practice that predates concepts of God and practices of religion, and consequently views all gods and belief systems with some degree of skepticism. Such things are relatively new and untested.

This is a practice of Yoga. Yoga unites body and mind, to strengthen both. Yoga is performed by Asanas, a fancy word for "resting." Just as sitting is a rest from standing, so is standing a rest from sitting; stillness rests from movement, movement from stillness. Go to Temple and come home; go home and go to work, go to work and then go play. There are millions of Asanas, and it is both impossible to practice them all, and ill advised to. Not all are suitable to your goals.

Hold not long enough, and you won't benefit. Hold too long, and you'll harm yourself – this you also shouldn't do. How long to hold an Asana? Svaha was the wife of Agni, a famous Yogi, who would practice so long his wife had to call him home: "you did it, sufficient, enough, success." Svaha! When Svaha calls to you, you have become like Agni. No, you have become Agni – this is the secret knowledge by which Yoga is learned.

Gain the second wind of athletic Indra and Kartekeya if you would be victorious. Bend the bow, bear the yoke, pull the plow, lift up the mountain, master time and space. Read minds - or know your own? Some Asanas are easier than others, some work is easier than others. But this does not make it any more right or wrong than what is difficult. But it does permit you to accomplish what is difficult. Free to do what is difficult or easy, you discover what is necessary and expedient.

This "necessary" is Dharma. Discover your Dharma, your nature, your duty. Knowing your duty, you won't hesitate to sacrifice what is required to accomplish it. Sacrificing for this necessary work becomes easier by practice, as any Asana does: sometimes it is necessary to work a difficult job, sacrificing for your family. Sometimes our duty is more difficult than this. Dharma permits work, Artha - by tirelessly working the Yogi learns that the benefits of this difficult work must be enjoyed if it is to be worthwhile, Kama. If something is necessary, Dharma, there will necessarily be benefit, Kama, from the sacrifice, and all effort, Artha, required for it.

A teenager attends to every strand of hair in a mirror before leaving the house: so should you exert self-control. In meditation we observe body, mind, thought, even self – self, our identity. We do not have souls or spirits - we do not believe in them. We have self, identify.

We develop awareness and insight for the purpose of self-improvement. Why self-improve? Because it is by self-control one becomes a Brahman, capable of sacrifice. Yoga is the literal "yoke" for this work. The Yogi holds the reins in self-restraint and bears the yoke, training so they may practice in improving their nature to perform their duty. Like Ganesh, the Yogi perfects their wisdom into contentment. Then, they can make a beginning of beginnings, and an ending of endings. Then they can sacrifice sacrificing. Jai Ganesh!

Let's begin a sacrifice? By Yoga one learns to give up, share, use up, exhaust. This is sacrifice! A book has a back cover: the Yogi puts it down when done. The teacher is surpassed – and year by year, millennia by millennia, we push the frontiers of the possible further, discovering our potential. And neither god nor religion nor any other triviality really is the purpose or the means of this exploration.

Our practice embraces belief and theology, even mysticism with its crystals and magic, understanding its importance for sacrifice into atheism and disbelief: what is laid down must be first taken up. But we then go beyond, to nontheism, we go far, far beyond belief.

We believe there are beliefs: these beliefs are taken up, then held onto. Even obsessed upon. Ignorance of truth creates a desire for belief, and this causes a hatred of what is contrary to that belief. We believe beliefs in this way cause distress. But beliefs can be let go of and uprooted.

Seeing is believing. Seeing is a belief. Hearing is a belief. Touching and tasting and smelling are all beliefs. Our perceptions are highly unreliable, shaped by biased thought, experience and incompetence. Bias! Through logic, through reason, we are able to understand better: there is no truth, there is no falsehood, there is only that which is not wholly untrue, not wholly false, that which is a little of both, and that which is not strictly speaking either. Such a world view requires detachment and abstraction:

though there is no such thing as a perfect square or circle, we can draw them to understand their relationships, and tolerate their imperfections. We construct counterfeit dharmas, training rules, and ritual. We learn to not pray. It is by strength and opportunity a Yogi fulfills their wishes.

But no, we are not Yogis. We have been for some recent years all of us "Hindus." And our rituals continue to strain against the nomenclature of a Christianity which cannot understand it. So our slogans, singing and training becomes an act of prayer, our lack of any god becomes a belief in the invisible god of the Judeo-Christian, our lifelong, devoted, loyal friendships become marriages, our freedom in society becomes caste by birth, and our lawlessness and immorality becomes barbaric, even wicked.

It is a fact we had no morality. So the Christian gave Hinduism morality, and the words to describe right and wrong. We had no religious leadership, no books of authority, no law – so we were given these too, and many illustrious Gurus and Swamis, that we would stop seeking the Priesthood which was our right. So much counterfeit dharma!

Yet this too is part of our Yoga: counterfeit dharma leads to a desire to let go of and sacrifice what is impure, inauthentic. This leads to take hold of what is authentic. And this then too is sacrificed, and let go of in its proper time and way. The purpose of practicing sacrifice is to sacrifice sacrificing.

The spectrum of Hinduism is practiced simultaneously, each individual accomplishing the Dharma. The Hindu slaughtering animals in sacrifice, whether on their dinner plate or on any other altar, is quite as Hindu as the Hindu sacrificing animals in an act of vegetarianism: all earn the same honor, performing an identical rite differently. None are more advanced nor primitive than the other. This same sacrifice is practiced in different ways, frequently for different goals. But with the same urgent necessity, the same Dharma. And with time, as we grow stronger and smarter, we learn the most expedient means to accomplish our goals. And what goals are most necessary. We learn what foods are more wholesome, how better to provide that food, and the purpose of gaining strength, and perpetuating our lives with food.

A Yogi cherishes their ritualized mysticism, even crystals and singing bowls. This is a rational and logical thing for any atheist to do if they will move beyond atheism to nontheism, and beyond nontheism by sacrifice.

I assure you, identification can be ceased. The suffering of identification can cease. And it must now cease. This is a call to sacrifice. Give up your beliefs, your identifications! Give up self, become selfless. Perform the self-sacrifice, and then begin Karma Yoga.

What is a Hindu? Am I a Hindu? Do I believe in God? I will tell you for someone who understands the Dharma, the question never arises even if I am man or woman? Or, am I anything at all? The question never arises, am I a Hindu? We do not attach to beliefs of such things as "I." Or "God." Not without the purpose of giving them up.

Translational notes and glossary

Translation is difficult, as the words convey concepts foreign to the culture and language of English. Often with subtle connotation. Consequently, to express understanding in this book, i have attempted to provide the means by which the reader can experience or come to understanding themselves, without the use of words. Below are presented several examples of the difficulty of providing a glossary, or definitions, in an apology to the reader if any terminology in this book proved challenging. Please contact the author through the publisher if you would better understand the intention of any word used in this book.

Dharma

Dharma: There is no single word definition for Dharma, but it does develop connotations of law, in the sense of natural laws of science: laws of physics, laws of economics, laws of humanity. Because of related conceptualizations, it is understood to connote what is proper, necessary, appropriate, or usually correct. In the sense that it is usually correct that a person may navigate by the north star (though exceptions are notable: this is not wholly an accurate understanding of "north" and cannot be used in the southern hemisphere, or with clouds, etc.): what is proper or necessary or appropriate or usually correct is not always so. From Dharma a concept of duty develops: in the sense of holding to principles of appropriateness (but being flexible in letting go of those principles). This holding (dhar/dar) can be understood by what is suitable, or fit. In the neo-Darwinian sense of fitness: survival of the sufficient (luck and opportunity play as much a role in survival as strength and intelligence): dharma is in this way understood by exploring in asanas "svaha," what is sufficient, successful, completed.

Asana

Asana: with the connotation of the seat of an elephant driver, or the military encampment of an occupying army posted against an enemy in that enemy's territory, the halt or rest in a military advance (in particular the last rest of annexation), or a dwelling where one sits (in the latin sense of sedes - a seat of power), or merely the non-martial necessity of sitting down to prevent or as a result of exhaustion and to recover strength, it is a compound form of "as" (presence, especially an aggressive assertion of that presence in close proximity, an urgent and exertive personal effort, and especially the exclamation of effort ("oh!" "ah!" "argh!" in English) and "ana" which means the breath or breathing (in the sense of "catching one's breath"). Together, this connotes aggression without malice - in the way that sports players will not hold malice against each other but still exert themselves fully, or an occupying army holds no malice to the new citizens being annexed, a needed rest or seat. In the sense that when one has stood too long, one must sit, or stand from sitting too long, finding rest in what action is easier to exert for what is difficult. Energetically, purposefully seeking and accomplishing rest.

Agni

Agni: the embodiment of the sacrificial fire or its heat, the stomach in the act of digestion or the gastric acids of digestion (in the sense that food is sacrificed by placing it into the burning/dissolving gastric fire by eating it), the color of fire (gold, not the metal, but the color), the abstract concept of "next." Or the conceptualization of the warmth of a room's the sunward exposure. It is also the abstract conceptualization of the matter of energy (energy and matter and force are all different concepts, which are basically the same in western scientific thinking). Also, the proper name of a deva

(deva is not "god" but "player," in an athletic or theatrical sense of the word who is renowned for sacrifices and yoga.

Indra

Indra: this is also the proper name of a deva (not a god, but player), but is better understood as a concept - one which is far too subtle and complex to adequately describe with succinctness. However, as an abstraction of "spirit" - in the sense of "athletic spirit," "heart" or "vigor" it may be understood in this context as the "igniter" of the fire (spark being necessary to fuel and air for combustion). In the understanding that the fire produces light as a benefit, and that a pupil is designed to accept that light (both the pupil of the eye and a pupil of a teacher). The pupil is what permits light to be seen (after shaped by the iris and lens) prior to being understood and controls all thought arising from that sensory organ ("seeing is believing"), in the understanding, that water may not be obstructed forever in its journey from sky to sea to sky again, Indra is the "King" of light, and belief (a form of maya). Indra is the second wind of an athlete, the recovery of strength after exhaustion or defeat, an unconquerable and indomitable freedom. Indra's primary "tool" is the vajra, a weaponized dart that symbolically represents a moment of time, a flash of understanding (like lightning), a strike or blow that brings victory by fulfilling the vow or purpose for the fighting (i.e. hatha yoga), success, victory. It is a weapon that is easily carried everywhere, easily mastered, and when tipped with glass or diamond, can control white light to separate the colors of the rainbow, revealing the composite nature of form, or pierce through any shielding, lie, illusion or other maya, and in this sense is partially symbolic of logic's power over belief. Indra connotes excellence, primacy, the first among equals, a subduer of challenge. As the lightning strike causes a wildfire that eventually burns itself out when it is "enough," accepting what is suitable, and rejecting what is not, Indra and Agni work together to complete a sacrifice.

Shanti

Shanti: the strength to remain undistressed against the action or presence of stressors, the ability to withstand aggression, or even change, the ability to conclude effort, whether successful or unsuccessful - peace.

Svaha